Violence and Psychopathy

Violence and Psychopathy

Edited by

Adrian Raine
Department of Psychology
University of Southern California
Los Angeles, California

José Sanmartín
Department of Logic and Philosophy of Science
University of Valencia
& Queen Sofia Center for the Study of Violence
Valencia, Spain

Kluwer Academic / Plenum Publishers
New York, Boston, Dordrecht, London, Moscow

Library of Congress Cataloging-in-Publication Data

Violencia y psicopatía. English
Violence and psychopathy/edited by Adrian Raine, José Sanmartín.
p. cm.
Previously published in Spanish: Barcelona: Editorial Ariel, 2000.
Includes bibliographical references and index.
ISBN 0-306-46669-4
1. Antisocial personality disorders. 2. Psychopaths. 3. Violence. 4. Deviant behavior. I. Raine, Adrian. II. Sanmartín, José, 1948– III. Centro Reina Sofía para el Estudio de la Violencia. IV. International Meeting on Biology and Sociology of Violence (4th: 1999: Valencia, Spain) V. Title.

RC555 .V5613 2001
616.85′82—dc21

2001038375

ISBN 0-306-46669-4

233 Spring Street, New York, New York 10013

http://www.wkap.nl/

10 9 8 7 6 5 4 3 2 1

A C.I.P. record for this book is available from the Library of Congress

Printed in the United States of America

CONTENTS

PREFACE

Adrian Raine
Department of Psychology, University of Southern California, USA

José Sanmartín
Queen Sofia Center for the Study of Violence, Valencia, Spain

The problems that psychopathic and violent offenders create for society are not restricted to North America. Instead, these offenders create havoc throughout the world, including Europe. In recognition of this fact, Queen Sophia of Spain has promoted a Center for the Study of Violence which recognizes both biological and social contributions to the cause of violence. In November 1999, the Queen Sofia Center for the Study of Violence held its IV International Meeting on the Biology and Sociology of Violence. This fourth Meeting, which was under the Honorary Presidency of H. M. The Queen of Spain, examined the biological, psychological and social aspects of the psychopath, the violent offender, and the serial killer. This book presents some of the key contributions made at that conference and which were first published in Spanish in 2000 by Ariel Press.

A key thrust of this book, and a stance shared by all of its contributors, is the notion that violence and psychopathy simply cannot be understood solely, or even fundamentally, in terms of social and environmental forces and influences. Nor do biological factors offer an exclusive explanation. Instead, it is likely that psychopathy is the result of complex interactions between biological and social factors, interactions which to date are poorly understood. Contributors to this book begin the difficult process of isolating the important biological, psychological, and social factors that contribute to violence. Once these factors are more fully understood, scientists will be in a better position to model their interactions and explain violence. The promise of such research is that ultimately we will be better placed to develop more effective intervention and prevention programs for violent and psychopathic offenders.

The first section of the book deals with psychopaths. In the United States, psychopaths are estimated to make up only 1% of the general public but as much as 25% of the prison population. According to a 1992 FBI study, 50%

of the law enforcement officers who died in the line of duty were killed by individuals who closely matched the personality profile of the psychopath. In addition, the reoffending rate of psychopaths is very high. Society's concept of the psychopath, shaped in part by the entertainment and news media, is that of a cold-blooded, remorseless predator who seeks, stalks, catches, tortures and murders his victims. But most psychopaths do not kill, and some of them to not commit any violence. Contributors to this book present a more data-based, rational analysis of the psychopathic offender with a particular focus on the neurobiological factors which shape psychopathy. By better understanding the mechanisms and processes that give rise to psychopathy, the belief is that we will be better placed to understand and control the wider problem of violence.

The second section deals with serial killers. Society tends to view serial killers as psychopaths, and there is certainly some justification for this view. Nevertheless, not all serial killers are psychopaths. Indeed, one contribution to this book divides serial killers into two categories: psychotics and psychopaths, with the latter predominating among those serial killers who plan their murders in cold blood, who are skilled at deceit and manipulation, and who stalk their victims. Yet another contribution provides a detailed analysis of the motivations of serial killers and the emotional meanings they attach to their life experiences.

The third section of the book deals with social contributions and treatment. Paradoxically, while we know much more about the social contributions to violence in general than we know about the biological contributions to violence, the reverse is true for psychopathy. That is, we know more about biological contributions to psychopathy than we know about social contributions. Nevertheless, this book includes contributions on social, psychological, and cognitive processes that play a role in shaping psychopathy. This book also deals with the elusive concept of the treatment of violence and psychopathy. There is increasing evidence that some treatment programs make psychopaths worse, i.e. they make them better-skilled psychopaths who are more likely to reoffend. Yet while we may not have any unquestionably effective treatment for psychopaths, it may be possible to identify components of programs that have been more successful than others, and to develop new programs that teach psychopaths cognitive skills that enable them to take more responsibility for their actions and to better meet their needs through non-criminal means.

Finally, we would like to acknowledge the invaluable help of the Queen Sofia Center for the Study of Violence in selecting, translating and correcting the various chapters of this book. We also wish to thank Andrea Macaluso of Kluwer/Plenum Publishers for her encouragement and helpful advice, and for seeing the value and contribution that this book can potentially make.

PART I

PSYCHOPATHS

Chapter 1

PSYCHOPATHS AND THEIR NATURE

Some Implications For Understanding Human Predatory Violence

Robert D. Hare
Department of Psychology, University of British Columbia, Vancouver, Canada

1. INTRODUCTION

In closing the "International Meeting on Biology and Sociology of Violence," held in Valencia in 1996, Her Majesty Queen Sophia of Spain noted that the future will see major advances in our understanding of—and our ability to deal with—the genetic and biological factors in aggression and violence. Her Majesty The Queen also offered the hope that the considerable information we already have concerning the environmental origins of violence would be put to more immediate use.

At the same meeting Eduardo Zaplana, President of the Community of Valencia, commented, "...specialists must diagnose, and with the knowledge provided, citizens and politicians must find solutions." And Dr. James S. Grisolía had this to say, "We misplace our focus on individual biology if we fail to recognize the interaction of the individual with his/her environment including other people...our social capacities are deeply ingrained in our biology."

Taken together, these cogent comments (published in Grisolía, Sanmartin, Luján, & Grisolía, 1997) serve to highlight several important premises for our efforts to understand the origins and use of human aggression and violence. First, aggression and violence are not unitary constructs. They take many forms and involve many levels of interpersonal and social complexity. The causes of violence at the interpersonal level are not the same as those that involve conflicts between groups or nations. Second, however we define aggression and violence, they are the result of exceedingly complex interactions between genetic/biological factors and social/environmental factors. It is unlikely that we soon will have more than a rudimentary grasp of these interactions, given our penchant for

Violence and Psychopathy, edited by Raine & Sanmartin,
Kluwer Academic/Plenum Publishers, New York, 2001.

investigating the two domains in isolation. Third, notwithstanding the importance of these interactions, we already know enough about the social and environmental correlates of individual and group violence to develop preventative strategies, given sufficient public pressure and political will. Fourth, we know relatively little about the biological bases of human violence, in part because of the complexity of the problems but also because until recently we lacked the investigative tools needed to provide basic information about the workings of the human brain. Fifth, it is unlikely that we ever will have a unified theory of violence. However, I believe that we now can see the modest beginnings of what might be referred to as a "mini-theory" of human predatory violence, based on the clinical and empirical research on psychopathy. This is the basis for my presentation. I will suggest that the aggression and violence of the psychopath are instrumental, predatory, and cold-blooded, and owe more to the nature of the individual than to the social and environmental forces that help to drive most other types of violence.

2. PSYCHOPATHY: THE CONCEPT

The modern conception of psychopathy is the result of several hundred years of clinical investigation and speculation by European and American psychiatrists and psychologists (see detailed accounts by Berrios, 1996; Millon, Simonsen, Birket-Smith, & Davis, 1998; McCord & McCord, 1964; Pichot, 1978). As Millon et al (1998) put it, "Psychopathy was the first personality disorder to be recognized in psychiatry. The concept has a long historical and clinical tradition, and in the last decade a growing body of research has supported its validity..." (p. 28). Although the etiology, dynamics, and conceptual boundaries of this personality disorder remain the subject of debate and research, there is a consistent clinical and empirical tradition concerning its core affective, interpersonal, and behavioral attributes. On the interpersonal level, psychopaths are grandiose, arrogant, callous, dominant, superficial, and manipulative. Affectively, they are short-tempered, unable to form strong emotional bond with others, and lacking in empathy, guilt or remorse. These interpersonal and affective features are associated with a socially deviant lifestyle that includes irresponsible and impulsive behavior, and a tendency to ignore or violate social conventions and mores.

Psychopathy cannot be understood solely, or even primarily, in terms of social and environmental forces and influences. It is likely that genetic factors contribute significantly to the personality traits and temperament considered essential to the disorder, although its lifelong expression is a product of complex interactions between biological/temperamental predispositions and social forces (Hare, 1993; Livesley, 1998). Certainly, the traits and behaviors that define adult psychopathy begin to manifest themselves early in childhood, in some cases as a combination of two diagnostic categories, conduct disorder and attention-deficit hyperactivity disorder (Frick, 1998; Lynam, 1966; McBride, 1998).

The biological and environmental mechanisms responsible for the development and maintenance of psychopathy are not well understood, though subject to much speculation (see Hare, 1993; Lykken, 1995; Mealey, 1995). Whether viewed as a mental disorder, a product of cerebral insult, an evolved "cheater" strategy for passing on one's gene pool (Mealey, 1995), or simply as a variant of normal personality (Widiger, 1998), psychopathy clearly presents society with a serious problem, as the rest of this chapter will attest. Although not all psychopaths come into formal contact with the criminal justice, their defining features clearly place them at high risk for aggression and violence. The problem, of course, is to identify these individuals as accurately as possible. This is particularly crucial in situations where a diagnosis of psychopathy has enormous implications for both the individual and society.

The importance of aggression and violence in psychopathic symptomatology has always been clear, and is well represented in current diagnostic criteria: those for antisocial personality disorder in the *Diagnostic and Statistical manual of mental Disorders* (DSM-IV; American Psychiatric Association, 1994); those for dyssocial personality in the *International Classification of Diseases and Related Health Problems* (ICD-10; World Health Organization, 1990); and those for psychopathy in the Hare Psychopathy Checklist-Revised (PCL-R; Hare, 1991). Each set contains one criterion directly related to a history of irritability, hostility, and aggression, including overt physical violence. In addition, each set contains several criteria that are indirectly related to aggression or violence (e.g., callousness, lack of remorse). It is worth noting that the historical link between psychopathy and violence is not peculiar to Western psychiatry. Indeed, psychopathy is a disorder that apparently occurs in every culture, and the potential for violence usually is considered symptomatic of the disorder (Cooke & Michie, 1999; Murphy, 1976).

Nevertheless, it is important to recognize that psychopathy is not synonymous with criminality. Most criminals are not psychopaths, and although all psychopaths violate many of society's rules and expectations, many probably manage to avoid formal contacts with the criminal justice system (see Hare, 1993). Some are unreliable and untrustworthy employees, unscrupulous and predatory businessmen, corrupt politicians, or unethical and amoral professionals whose prestige and power are used to victimize their clients, patients, and the general public. Except for occasional media coverage and anecdotal clinical reports, we know little about these individuals. Systematic research is needed to determine the prevalence of psychopathy in the general population, the varieties of criminal and noncriminal ways in which the disorder manifests itself, and the extent to which research with criminal psychopaths informs us about psychopaths in general. With respect to the latter issues, there are indications that the personality structure and propensity for unethical behavior probably are much the same in criminal and noncriminal (or "subcriminal") psychopaths (e.g., Babiak, 1995; Cleckley, 1976; Forth, Brown, Hart, & Hare, 1996; Gustafson & Ritzer, 1995; Hare, 1993).

Following a brief description of current assessment procedures, I will devote the remainder of this presentation to the association between psychopathy and the propensity for predatory violence, and to some possible neurobiological correlates of this propensity.

3. THE ASSESSMENT OF PSYCHOPATHY

Two major approaches to the assessment of psychopathy have influenced current clinical practice and empirical research, particularly in North America and, increasingly, in Europe. One is reflected in the DSM-III,-III-R, and -IV criteria for antisocial personality disorder, and is based in part on the assumptions that it is difficult for clinicians to assess personality traits reliably, and that early-onset delinquency is a cardinal symptom of the disorder (Robins, 1978). These assumptions account for the heavy emphasis on delinquent and antisocial behavior in the criteria set for antisocial personality disorder (Hare & Hart, 1995; Widiger et al, 1996; Widiger & Corbitt, 1995).

The other approach stems naturally from a rich European and North American clinical tradition reflected, for example, in the writings of Cleckley (1976), the ICD-10 diagnostic criteria for dysocial personality disorder, and in the efforts of researchers to provide a sound conceptual and psychometric basis for assessing the disorder. This traditional conception of psychopathy has been operationalized in the Hare PCL-R and its derivatives, including a screening version (PCL:SV) and a youth version (PCL:YV) of the PCL-R. The rationale for the PCL-R is that assessment must be based on the full range of psychopathic symptomatology. A focus on antisocial behaviors, to the exclusion of interpersonal and affective symptoms (e.g., callousness, grandiosity, deceitfulness, lack of empathy), leads to the overdiagnosis of psychopathy in criminal populations and to underdiagnosis in noncriminals. In this respect, the PCL-R is made up of two correlated clusters of features, or factors. Factor 1 reflects the interpersonal and affective components of the disorder, whereas Factor 2 is more closely allied with a socially deviant lifestyle. I might note here that the DSM-IV category, antisocial personality disorder, is strongly associated with PCL-R Factor 2, but only weakly associated with Factor 1.

Items in the Hare Psychopathy Checklist-Revised (PCL-R)

Factor 1: Interpersonal/affective	Factor 2: Social Deviance
1. Glibness/superficial charm	3. Need for stimulation/proneness to boredom
2. Grandiose sense of self worth	9. Parasitic lifestyle
4. Pathological lying	10. Poor behavioral controls
5. Conning/manipulative	12. Early behavioral problems
6. Lack of remorse or guilt	13. Lack of realistic, long-term goals
7. Shallow affect	14. Impulsivity
8. Callous/lack of empathy	15. Irresponsibility
16. Failure to accept responsibility for own actions	18. Juvenile delinquency
	19. Revocation of conditional release
*Additional Items	
11. Promiscuous sexual behavior	17. Many short-term marital relationships
20. Criminal versatility	

Note: From Hare (1991). The rater uses specific criteria, interview and file information to score each item on a 3-point scale (0, 1, 2).
* Items that do not load on either factor.

Table 1. Items in the Hare Psychopathy Checklist-Revised (PCL-R)

To ensure accurate diagnosis the PCL-R uses expert observer (i.e., clinical) ratings, based on a semi-structured interview, a review of case history materials—such as criminal or psychiatric records, interviews with family members and employers, and so forth—and supplemented with behavioral observations whenever possible. Specific scoring criteria are used to rate each of 20 items on a 3-point scale (0, 1, 2) according to the extent to which it applies to a given individual. Total scores can range from 0 to 40 and reflect the degree to which the individual matches the prototypical psychopath. The mean score is about 22-24 (SD about 7-8) in offender populations and about 18-20 (SD about 7-8) in forensic psychiatric populations. A score of 30 typically is used as a diagnostic cutoff for psychopathy, although some investigators adopt less stringent cutoffs for certain populations (see below). PCL-R assessments are highly reliable and valid when made by qualified clinicians and researchers. Indeed, Fulero (1995) described the PCL-R as the "state of the art...both clinically and in research use." Although developed primarily with data from male offenders and forensic patients, the psychometric properties of the PCL-R now are well established in a variety of other offender and patient populations, including females, adolescents, substance abusers, and sex offenders. The empirical work discussed in the rest of this presentation was based on the use of the PCL-R or its derivatives (a list of publications with the PCL-R and its derivatives can be found on my web site, www.hare.org).

Research indicates that the PCL-R also has good cross-cultural generalizability (Cooke, 1998; Cooke & Michie, 1999; Hare, Clark, Grann, & Thornton, 2000). Moreover, Cooke and his colleagues have used item response theory (IRT), also known as latent trait theory, to investigate the discriminating properties of the PCL-R and PCL:SV items. IRT provides information about the extent to which individual items (or groups of items) are discriminating of (or relevant to) a given construct or trait, in this case, psychopathy. They found that the interpersonal and affective (Factor 1) items are more discriminating of the psychopathy construct, or latent trait, than are the socially deviant (Factor 2) items (Cooke & Michie, 1997; Cooke, Michie, Hart, & Hare, 1999). Recently, Cooke and Michie (in press) used IRT and reanalysis of several large sets of PCL-R data to argue that psychopathy can better be viewed as a superordinate construct consisting of 13 PCL-R items that cluster into three factors: interpersonal, affective, and lifestyle. The first two factors represent a split of PCL-R Factor 1 into two parts, while the third factor is derived from PCL-R Factor 2.

4. PSYCHOPATHY AND CRIME

In the past few years there has been a dramatic change in the role played by psychopathy in the criminal justice system. Formerly, a prevailing view was that clinical diagnoses of psychopathy were of little value in understanding and predicting criminal behaviors. However, even a cursory inspection of the features that define the disorder –callousness, impulsivity, egocentricity, grandiosity, irresponsibility, lack of empathy, guilt, or remorse, and so forth– indicates that psychopaths should be much more likely than other members of the general public to bend and break the rules and laws of society. Although there never has been a shortage of anecdotal reports and clinical speculations about the association between psychopathy and crime, the widespread adoption of the PCL-R as a common metric has provided robust empirical evidence on this.

Although psychopathy is closely associated with antisocial and criminal behavior, psychopaths are qualitatively different from others who routinely engage in criminal behavior, different even from those whose criminal conduct is extremely serious and persistent. The typical criminal career is relatively short, but there are individuals who devote most of their adolescent and adult life to delinquent and criminal activities. Among these persistent offenders are psychopaths, who begin their antisocial and criminal activities at a relatively early age, and continue to engage in these activities throughout much of the life span. Many of these "career" criminals become less grossly antisocial in middle age. About half of the criminal psychopaths we have studied show a relatively sharp reduction in criminality around age 35 or 40 (Hare, McPherson, & Forth, 1988). This does not mean that they have given up crime completely, only that their level of general criminal activity has decreased to that of the average persistent offender. Moreover, this age-related decrease in crime may not apply to violent acts. The propensity for psychopaths to engage in violent and aggressive behavior appears to decrease very little with age.

5. PSYCHOPATHY AND PREDATORY VIOLENCE

Many of the characteristics important for inhibiting antisocial and violent behavior –empathy, close emotional bonds, fear of punishment, guilt– are lacking or seriously deficient in psychopaths. Moreover, their egocentricity, grandiosity, sense of entitlement, impulsivity, general lack of behavioral inhibitions, and need for power and control, constitute what might be described as the perfect prescription for asocial, antisocial, and criminal acts. This would help to explain why psychopaths make up only about 1% of the general population but as much as a quarter of our prison populations. It also would explain why they find it so easy to victimize the vulnerable and to use intimidation and violence as tools to achieve power and control over others. As Silver, Mulvey, & Monahan (1999) put it, "Psychopathy's defining characteristics, such as impulsivity, criminal versatility, callousness, and lack of empathy or remorse make the conceptual link between violence and psychopathy straightforward" (p. 244).

Many of the attitudes and behaviors of psychopaths have a predatory quality about them. Psychopaths apparently see others as little more than emotional, physical, and financial prey, and feel justified in their belief that the world is made up of "givers and takers" and that they are "natural born takers." They are skilled at camouflage (deception, manipulation), stalking, and locating life's "feeding grounds" and "watering holes." Moreover, their use of intimidation and violence tends to be cold-blooded and instrumental (e.g., Cornell et al, 1996), and is more likely to be straightforward, uncomplicated, and businesslike ("a matter of process") than an expression of deep-seated distress or understandable precipitating factors. It lacks the emotional coloring that characterizes the violence of most other individuals. The reactions of psychopaths to the damage they have inflicted are more likely to be cool indifference, a sense of power, pleasure, or smug satisfaction than regret or concern for what they have done. The ease with which psychopaths engage in violence has very real significance for society in general and for law enforcement personnel in particular. For example, a study by the Federal Bureau of Investigation (1992) found that almost half of the law enforcement officers who died in the line of duty were killed by individuals, mostly strangers, who closely matched the personality profile of the psychopath. And perhaps as many as 25-30% of persistent wife-batterers in court-mandated treatment programs may be psychopaths (e.g., see Dutton & Kropp, 2000).

6. PSYCHOPATHY AND THE PREDICTION OF VIOLENCE

Until recently, a common view was that personality traits and clinical diagnoses added little to understanding and predicting criminal and violent behaviors. This implies that two offenders with the same scores on some actuarial device –based on similar criminal and demographic characteristics– should have the same risk for reoffending, even though one is an egocentric, cold-blooded, and remorseless psychopath while the other is not. Logically, they should not present the same risk. And empirically, they do not, particularly with respect to violence.

The significance of psychopathy as a robust risk factor for recidivism in general, and for violence in particular, is now well established (see meta-analyses by Dolan & Doyle, 2000; Salekin, Rogers, & Sewell, 1996; Hemphill, Hare, & Wong, 1998). In their review, Salekin et al (1996) concluded that the ability of the PCL-R to predict violence was "unparalleled" and "unprecedented" in the literature on the assessment of dangerousness. Although a detailed account of psychopathy as a risk for recidivism and violence is beyond the scope of this presentation, some examples may be helpful.

6.1. Adult Offenders

In the first prospective study of its type (Hart, Kropp, & Hare, 1988), we administered the PCL-R to 231 male offenders prior to their conditional release from a federal prison, and then followed their progress in the community for up to approximately 40 months or until "failure," defined as a return to prison because of a new offence or a violation of the terms of the conditional release. Multiple regression analyses indicated that the PCL-R made a significant contribution to the prediction of failure, over and above the contribution made by relevant criminal-history and demographic variables. Because we were interested when the first failure occurred, we subjected the data to a survival analysis in which survival –that is, not being returned to prison– was calculated as a function of time following release. By the end of the study period 81% of the offenders with high PCL-R scores had failed, compared with a failure rate of 62% for those with medium PCL-R scores and 29% for those with low PCL-R scores.

Similar results have been obtained by other investigators. For example, Hodgins, Cote, and Ross (1992) administered the French version of the PCL-R to 97 male offenders prior to their release on parole, and followed their progress for up to one year. The failure rate for offenders with high, medium, and low PCL-R scores was approximately 60%, 40%, and 10%, respectively.. Serin and Amos (1995) administered the PCL-R to 299 male offenders and followed them for up to eight years. The failure rate for those with high, medium, and low PCL-R scores was 80%, 62%, and 29%, respectively. Interestingly, the rate for *violent* reoffending in this sample was about 40% for those with a high PCL-R score but only about 10% for the other offenders..

The role of psychopathy in the prediction of violence is impressive. When measured by the PCL-R or its derivatives, it frequently is the *best* predictor. Harris, Rice, and Quinsey (1993) found that the PCL-R was the single most important predictor of violent recidivism in a large sample of offenders released from a maximum security unit and a pretrial assessment center. In a Swedish study, Grann, Langström, Tengström, and Kullgren (1999) evaluated the relationship between the PCL-R and violent reoffending in a sample of 352 personality disordered offenders released into the community. They found that risk for violent recidivism during a follow-up period that averaged more than four years was about 68%for offenders with a high PCL-R score,, 50% for those with a medium score, and 24% for those with a low PCL-R score. Grann et al (1999) also performed a receiver operating characteristic (ROC) analysis of the PCL-R and violent recidivism. The ROC curve is a plot of true positives (sensitivity) against false positives (1 minus specificity), and is independent of the base rate for violence. The area under the curve (AUC; the area between the curve and the diagonal) represents the probability that a violent patient will have a higher PCL-R score than will a nonviolent patient. The AUC was .67 within 6 months, .71 within 1 year, and .70 within 5 years following release. They concluded that the PCL-R was as valid a predictor of violent recidivism in Swedish forensic settings as it is in North American settings, a conclusion that held whether or not the offenders were born in Sweden, and even after other risk factors were taken into account.

Relatively little research has been conducted on psychopathy in adult female offenders. However, the available data indicate that, on average, about 15% of female offenders meet the PCL-R criteria for psychopathy (Hemphill, Strachan, & Hare, 1999). The recidivism rate for these offenders is considerably higher than it is for other female offenders. For example, in one study (see Hemphill et al, 1999) about 60% of the female psychopaths reoffended within one year of release, compared with less than 20% of the nonpsychopaths. Salekin, Rogers, Ustad, & Sewell (1998) reported that at 50 days following release from prison the recidivism rate for female psychopaths was almost seven times the rate for other female offenders. However, after 50 days the difference between the groups disappeared. Loucks & Zamble (2000) found that in a sample of 100 female offenders the PCL-R was strongly associated with total criminal convictions (r = .49), violent criminal convictions (r = .46), institutional infractions (r = .63), and violent institutional infractions (r = .38). The PCL-R also was a strong predictor of recidivism in this study (E. Zamble, personal communication, February, 2001). Thus, within four years of release, the reconviction rate of offenders with high, medium, and low PCL-R scores was 79%, 40%, and 22%, respectively.

6.2. Adolescent Offenders

Psychopathy does not emerge unannounced in adulthood. As I've indicated above, the precursors are apparent at an early age, and the disorder can be measured reliably with the PCL:YV (Forth & Burke, 1998; Forth et al, in press) in adolescence. The base rate of psychopathy is at least as high among adolescent offenders as among their adult counterparts. These adolescent psychopaths are at much higher risk for recidivism and violence than are other adolescent offenders. In one study, Gretton (1998) examined the predictive validity of the PCL:YV in a large sample of young offenders, age 12 to 18, who had been sent by the courts to a youth facility for presentence psychological and psychiatric evaluation. In the 10-year follow-up period, the psychopaths were much more likely to violently reoffend than were the other adolescents. Even when relevant demographic and criminal history variables were taken into account, the PCL:YV made a substantial and significant contribution to the prediction of violent offending. In fact, a history of violence was unrelated to subsequent violence, both in psychopaths and nonpsychopaths. That is, offenders with no prior evidence of violence were just as likely to commit a violent offence during the follow-up period as were those with a history of violence.

Forth, Hart, & Hare (1990) administered an early version of the PCL:YV to a sample of high risk adolescent offenders in a maximum-security facility. Forth (1995) reported that subsequent to their release into the community the psychopaths, now approaching early adulthood, committed almost four times as many violent crimes as did the other offenders. Toupin Mercier, Déry, Côté, & Hodgins (1996) administered a French translation of the PCL-R (see Côté & Hodgins, 1996) to male adolescents receiving treatment in rehabilitation centers, day centers, or special educational programs. During a 1-year follow-up period, PCL-R scores were significantly correlated with delinquency, aggressive behavior, alcohol use, and number of aggressive conduct disorder symptoms. Similar results were obtained by Brandt, Kennedy, Patrick, and Curtin (1997) with a sample of mostly African-American young offenders. In a recent review, Edens, Skeem, Cruise, and Cauffman (2001) concluded that the PCL-R and its modification, the PCL:YV, had much the same association with aggressive behavior as that found with adult offenders.

6.3. Forensic Psychiatric Patients

The prevalence of psychopathy, as measured by the PCL-R or PCL:SV, is somewhat lower in forensic psychiatric populations (about 10-15%) than it is in prison populations (about 15-25%). However, forensic patients who meet the criteria for psychopathy or who have a significant number of psychopathic traits are at much higher risk for recidivism and violence than are other forensic patients. For example, several studies have found that psychopathy is predictive of institutional aggression and violence in forensic psychiatric hospitals (Hill, Rogers, & Bickford, 1996; Heilbrun et. al., 1998). Rice and Harris (1992) found that scores on the PCL-R were as predictive of recidivism in a sample of male not-guilty-by-reason-of-insanity (NGRI) schizophrenics as in a sample of nonpsychotic offenders. Hart and Hare (1989) found that only a small minority of consecutive admissions to a forensic psychiatric hospital were psychopaths, but that many patients exhibited a significant number of PCL-R symptoms. Further, the PCL-R predicted recidivism rates in a 5-year follow-up period (Wintrup, 1994).

A recent Swedish study (Tengström, Grann, Langström, & Kullgren, 2000) illustrates that there is a strong association between psychopathy and violence even in forensic patients with a history of violence. The sample in this study consisted of 202 violent psychotic offenders (most of whom were schizophrenics) with a mean PCL-R score of 18.2 (SD = 7.5). Patients with a PCL-R score above 25 (psychopaths; about 22% of the sample) were about four times more likely to violently recidivate in the post-release follow-up period (which averaged 51 months) than were those with a PCL-R score of 25 or below. A set of established risk factors for this population could not improve on the predictive power of the PCL-R. Moreover, PCL-R Factor 1 (interpersonal/affective features) was as predictive of violence as was Factor 2 (socially deviant lifestyle). An additional finding of note was a sharp increase in the likelihood of a violent offence shown by the psychopaths at about 48 months post-release. Apparently this coincided with the end of intensive community supervision, suggesting that tight supervision is a protective factor for psychopaths. An ROC analysis obtained an AUC of .75 for the PCL:SV and violent recidivism within five years.

6.4. Civil Psychiatric Patients

The relationship between psychopathy and the prediction of violence is not confined to prison and forensic psychiatric populations. Several recent studies clearly indicate that the PCL:SV is one of the strongest risk factors for violence in civil psychiatric patients.

In one study, Douglas, Ogloff, & Nicholls (1997) assessed post-release community violence in a sample of 167 male and 112 female patients who had been involuntarily committed to a civil psychiatric facility. Although very few of the patients had a score high enough to warrant a diagnosis of psychopathy, the PCL:SV nevertheless was highly predictive of violent behaviors and arrests for violent crimes. When the distribution of PCL:SV scores was split at the median (about 8 on a scale of 0-24), the odds ratio for an arrest for violent crime was about 10 times higher for patients above the median than it was for those below the median. The results of an ROC analysis of the PCL:SV and violent arrests yielded an AUC of .75.

In the MacArthur Foundation's Violence Risk Assessment Study, the most extensive and thorough study of its sort ever conducted, 134 potential predictors of violence in 939 patients were evaluated over a 20-week period following discharge from a civil psychiatric facility (Steadman et al, 2000). The single best predictor was the PCL:SV. The prevalence of post-discharge violence was 35.7% for patients with a PCL:SV score of 13 or more (out of a maximum of 24), but only 12.6% for patients with a PCL:SV score of less than 13. In presenting their results, the authors used a "classification tree" approach in which a hierarchy of decisions is made about the risk posed by a given patient. In this scheme, the first decision is whether or not the patient has a PCL:SV score of 13 or more. Silver, Mulvey, and Monahan (1999) used a subsample of 293 of these patients to investigate the impact that neighborhood factors have on individual risk factors for violence in discharged patients. Again, the single best predictor of violence was the PCL:SV; the odds that a patient with a PCL:SV score of 13 or more would commit a violent act were 5.3 times higher than were the odds that a patient with a score below 13 would commit such an act. Although patients discharged into neighborhoods with "concentrated poverty" generally were at higher risk for violence than were those discharged into neighborhoods with less poverty, the odds ratio for psychopathy associated with violence changed very little (from 5.3 to 4.8) when concentrated poverty was added to the equation.

6.5. Sexual Violence

The last few years have seen a sharp increase in public and professional attention paid to sex offenders, particularly those who commit a new offense following release from a treatment program or prison. It has long been recognized that psychopathic sex offenders present special problems for therapists and the criminal justice system. For example, the Kansas Sexually Violent Predator Act established procedures for the involuntary commitment of sexually violent predators, defined as "any person who has been convicted of or charged with a sexually violent offense and who suffers from a mental abnormality or personality disorder which makes the person likely to engage in the predatory acts of sexual violence." In a landmark decision (Kansas vs. Hendricks, June, 1997), the United States Supreme Court upheld the constitutionality of such an involuntary commitment. As a result, many States are now introducing legislation that will allow for the civil commitment of dangerous sex offenders following their release from prison. Because most of these individuals will be psychopaths, Tucker (1999) has argued that the Supreme Court's decision will result in mixing the "bad" with the "mad," psychopathic criminals with psychiatric patients.

Several studies have investigated the prevalence of psychopathy among various types of sex offenders (e.g., Brown & Forth, 1997; Miller, Geddings, Levenston, and Patrick, 1994; Porter, Fairweather, Drugge, Hervé, Birt, & Boer, 2000; Quinsey, Rice, & Harris, 1995). In general, the prevalence of psychopathy, as measured by the PCL-R, is much lower in child molesters (around 10-15%) than in rapists or "mixed" offenders (around 40-50%). The offences of psychopathic sex offenders are likely to be more violent or sadistic than are those of other sex offenders (Barbaree, Seto, Serin, Amos, and Preston, 1994; Brown and Forth, 1997; Firestone, Bradford, & Larose, 1998; Miller et al, 1994; Serin, Malcolm, Khanna, & Barbaree, 1994). In extreme cases –for example, among serial killers– comorbidity of psychopathy and sadistic personality is very high (Stone, 1998).

6.6. A Potent Combination

Sex offenders generally are resistant to treatment, but it is the psychopaths among them who are most likely to recidivate early and often. Quinsey et al. (1995) concluded that psychopathy functions as a general predictor of sexual and violent recidivism. They found that within 6 years of release from prison more than 80% of the psychopaths, but only about 20% of the nonpsychopaths, had violently recidivated. Many, but not all, of their offenses were sexual in nature.

One of the most potent combinations to emerge from the recent research on sex offenders is psychopathy, coupled with evidence of deviant sexual arousal. In a recent follow-up of a large sample of sex offenders, Rice and Harris (1997) reported that the PCL-R was highly predictive of violent recidivism in general. In addition, however, they found that sexual recidivism (as opposed to violent recidivism in general) was strongly predicted by a combination of a high PCL-R score and phallometric evidence of deviant sexual arousal, defined as any phallometric test that indicated a preference for deviant stimuli, such as children, rape cues, or nonsexual violence cues. Similarly, Harris & Hanson (1998) reported that offenders with a high PCL-R score and behavioral evidence of sexual deviance had committed more pre-index sexual offences, more kidnapping and forcible confinements, and more general (nonsexual) offences, and were more likely to violently recidivate, than were other offenders.

The implications of psychopathy and deviant sexual arousal appear to be as serious among adolescent sex offenders as among their adult counterparts. Gretton, McBride, Hare, O'Shaughnessy, & Kumka, in press) tracked the criminal activities of a large sample of adolescent sex offenders for five years following their release from a sex-offender treatment facility. The reconviction rate for sexual and other violent offences in the first 5 years following release was more than three times greater for those with a high PCL:YV score than it was for those with a low PCL:YV score. A high PCL:YV score and phallometric evidence of deviant sexual arousal was associated with a high risk for general and violent reoffending. The difference between these results and those obtained with adult sex offenders (Rice & Harris, 1997) is that the combination of psychopathy and deviant arousal was predictive of sexual violence in adults, whereas it was predictive of general offending, including violence, in adolescents. It is possible that as these adolescent offenders age the combination of psychopathy and deviant sexual arousal will become less predictive of offending in general, and more predictive of sexual offending in particular.

In any case, it is likely that many sex offenders, and most psychopathic ones, are more likely to be convicted of a nonsexual than a sexual offense. Many of these individuals are not so much specialized sex offenders as they are general, versatile offenders. Their misbehavior –sexual and otherwise– presumably is a reflection of factors not specifically related to sexual behavior. For the psychopaths, these factors no doubt include their personality structure, their predatory stance, and their readiness to take advantage of any opportunities that come their way. It may be more important to target the antisocial tendencies and behaviors of so-called psychopathic sex offenders than it is to treat their sexual deviancy.

7. TREATMENT OF PSYCHOPATHS

There is little convincing scientific evidence that psychopaths respond favorably to treatment and intervention (see Dolan & Coid, 1993; Hare, 1993; Losel, 1998; Suedfeld & Landon, 1978). This does not mean that their attitudes and behaviors are immutable, only that there have been no methodologically sound treatment or "resocialization" programs that have been shown to work with psychopaths.

Several empirical studies illustrate the point. For example, Ogloff, Wong, and Greenwood (1990) reported that psychopaths, defined by a PCL-R score of at least 30, derived little benefit from a therapeutic community program designed to treat personality-disordered offenders. The psychopaths stayed in the program for a shorter time, were less motivated, and showed less clinical improvement than did other offenders. It might be argued that even though the psychopaths did not do well in this program, some residual benefits could conceivably show up following their release from prison. However, in a survival analysis Hemphill (1991) found that the estimated reconviction rate in the first year following release was twice as high for the psychopaths as for the other offenders. Rice, Harris, and Cormier (1992) retrospectively scored the PCL-R from the institutional files of patients of a maximum security psychiatric facility. They defined psychopaths by a PCL-R score of 25 or more, and nonpsychopaths by a score below 25. They then compared the violent recidivism rate of patients who had been treated in an intensive and lengthy therapeutic community program with patients who had not taken part in the program. For nonpsychopaths, the violent recidivism rate of treated patients was half that of untreated patients. But the violent recidivism rate of treated psychopaths was about 50% higher than that of untreated psychopaths. Therapy apparently made the psychopaths worse. But why? The simple answer is that group therapy and insight-oriented programs may help psychopaths to develop better ways of manipulating, deceiving, and using people, but do little to help them to understand themselves. As a consequence, following release into the community they may be more likely than untreated psychopaths to continue to place themselves in situations where the potential for violence is high.

The findings by Rice et al. (1992), though intriguing and suggestive, were based on retrospective research with a particular population of mentally disordered offenders, and with an unusual, complex, and highly controversial treatment program that included the use of LSD and nude-encounter therapy. These problems notwithstanding, there is recent evidence that psychopaths are not good candidates for traditional forms of prison treatment. Hobson, Shine, and Roberts (2000) administered the PCL-R to patients when they entered an English prison hospital for treatment in a well-developed therapeutic community program. Their behavior during treatment sessions and while on the wards was evaluated with specially designed checklists. High scores on the PCL-R were strongly predictive of disruptive behaviors during treatment sessions and on the wards 3 months and 6 months following admission to the prison. The effect was entirely due to the interpersonal and affective features of psychopathy (PCL-R Factor 1). The results clearly indicated that the psychopaths manipulated the system to satisfy their own need for power, control, and prestige. They played "head games" with other inmates and staff, continually tested the boundaries and looked for people and things to exploit, and showed no genuine interest in changing their own attitudes and behavior. Nevertheless, they managed to manipulate and fool some staff into thinking their efforts were sincere and that they were making good progress.

A recent analysis of outcome in the English Prison Service (Hare, Clark, Grann, & Thornton, 2000) indicated that various short-term treatment programs, including educational upgrading and the development of social skills, had little effect on the post-release recidivism rates of offenders with low or moderate PCL-R scores. However, these same programs appear to *increase* the post-release recidivism rates of offenders with high PCL-R scores. The effect was particularly strong when offenders were divided on the basis of their score on Factor 1 of the PCL-R. Thus, the two-year post-release recidivism rate for those with a low Factor 1 score was 31% for those who had participated in a prison treatment program and 32% if they had not done so. In sharp contrast, the recidivism rate for offenders with a high Factor 1 score was 58% if they had not taken part in a prison treatment program, but 85% if they had.

In many respects, findings of this sort are understandable. Unlike most other offenders, psychopaths appear to suffer little personal distress, see little wrong with their attitudes and behavior, and seek treatment only when it is in their best interests to do so, such as when seeking probation or parole. It is therefore not surprising that they derive little benefit from traditional prison programs, particularly those aimed at the development of empathy, conscience, and interpersonal skills. What then? Do we simply keep them in prison until they are old enough to pose little risk to society? Do we ask psychopaths to participate in treatment programs that have little chance of success and that fool them and us into thinking that the exercise is worthwhile and of practical benefit to them? Rather than being discouraged, we should mount a concerted effort to develop innovative procedures designed specifically for psychopathic offenders.

Lösel (1998) has provided a thoughtful analysis of the issues involved in the treatment and management of psychopathic and other offenders, and has outlined in some detail the requirements for an effective program. An extensive set of program guidelines for development of a program specifically designed for psychopaths is now available (Wong & Hare, in press). In brief, we propose that relapse-prevention techniques should be integrated with elements of the best available cognitive-behavioral correctional programs. The program is less concerned with developing empathy and conscience or effecting changes in personality than with convincing participants that they alone are responsible for their behavior, and that they can learn more prosocial ways of using their strengths and abilities to satisfy their needs and wants. It involves tight control and supervision, both in the institution and following release into the community, as well as comparisons with carefully selected groups of offenders treated in standard correctional programs. The experimental design would permit empirical evaluation of its treatment and intervention modules (what works and what doesn't work for particular individuals). That is, some modules or components might be effective with psychopaths but not with other offenders, and vice versa. Because correctional programs are constantly in danger of erosion because of changing institutional priorities, community concerns, and political pressures, we proposed stringent safeguards for maintaining the integrity of the program.

8. SOME NEUROBIOLOGICAL HYPOTHESES AND RESEARCH

It is clear from the preceding review that psychopaths apparently have little or no compunction about using violence to attain their goals. As I've written elsewhere (Hare, 1998), even experienced clinicians and researchers often are stunned by the apparent ease with which these individuals engage in cold-blooded, instrumental behavior. They also are puzzled by the candid — yet obviously superficial and mechanical — manner in which many of these individuals describe their actions, their feelings about what they have done, and the impact their behavior might have had on others. Their expressions of remorse are accepted at face value by some people, but astute observers find their words unconvincing, little more than mimicry of something poorly understood.

Some psychopaths are perfectly frank about their inability to understand or experience what others describe as intense emotional feelings. In a book about his experiences in prison, a convicted killer wrote, "There are emotions—a whole spectrum of them—that I know only through words, through reading and in my immature imagination. I can imagine I feel these emotions but I do not" (see Hare, 1993, pp. 42-43). With the help of several prominent people he secured his release from prison and impulsively stabbed to death an unarmed waiter during an argument about a trivial matter. The depth of his emotional concern for the man he had killed, an aspiring actor, is apparent from the following remarks, *"There was no pain, it was a clean wound....He had no future as an actor — chances are he would have gone into another line of work."* Here we have an otherwise intelligent man who describes an impulsive killing in a dispassionate, matter-of-fact manner, and who cannot comprehend what the fuss is all about. To say that there is something unusual about people like him is an understatement. While the cognitions and interpersonal interactions of most members of our species are heavily laden with emotion (Damasio, 1994), those of psychopaths seem shallow and emotionally barren. Moreover, their behaviors often have a disinhibitory (impulsive, unrestrained) quality about them. The question is, why?

Although we are a long way from having all the answers, the increasing use of procedures and paradigms from cognitive psychology and neuroscience is beginning to provide some interesting clues. I've discussed much of this research in detail elsewhere (Hare, 1998), and will focus here on some recent applications of electrocortical and neuroimaging technology to the problem of psychopathy. What I have to say nicely complements the theoretical and empirical work by Christopher Patrick on emotional processing, and by Adrian Raine on the role of the frontal cortex in criminal and violent behavior.

The starting point for my discussion is the evidence that psychopaths fail to appreciate the emotional significance of an event or experience (Hare, 1978; Intrator et al., 1997; Patrick, 1994; Williamson, Harpur, & Hare, 1991). Although not confined to linguistic processes, it is their use of language that most clearly illustrates what is "wrong" with psychopaths (cf., Cleckley, 1976). It appears that they are unable or unwilling to process or use the deep semantic and affective meanings of language. Their linguistic processes are relatively superficial, and the subtle, more abstract meanings and nuances of language seem to escape them (Cleckley, 1976; Gillstrom, 1995; Hare, 1993; Intrator et al., 1997; Williamson et al, 1991). In short, psychopaths appear to be semantically and affectively shallow individuals, a conclusion that follows naturally from both clinical and laboratory work.

We might speculate that the deep semantic and affective networks that tie cognitions together are not well developed in psychopaths, for reasons that are not yet clear. One possibility is that the cognitive, linguistic, and behavioral attributes of psychopaths are related to an unusual inter-hemispheric distribution of processing resources (see discussions by Hare, 1998; Kosson & Harpur, 1997). It is also possible that the disorder involves some form of cerebral dysfunction, particularly in frontal cortex (Gorenstein & Newman, 1980; Hare, 1998; Intrator et al., 1997; Kiehl, Hare, McDonald, & Brink, 1999; Lapierre, Braun, & Hodgins, 1995; Liddle, Smith, Kiehl, Mendrek, & Hare, 1999; Raine, 1996). If so, the damage must be rather subtle, given that psychopaths often perform normally on standard neuropsychological tests, including those that reflect frontal functions (Hare, 1991; Hart, Forth, & Hare, 1990). This does not necessarily mean that a brain dysfunction model is untenable, only that the abnormality may be more functional than structural, in which case it would be fruitful to employ the sorts of information-processing tasks used in cognitive neuroscience, particularly in conjunction with psychophysiological procedures and neuroimaging technology. Such an approach would allow us to investigate the manner in which psychopaths might differ from others in the use of cognitive strategies, and in the structural and functional mechanisms and circuits that underlie their cognitions, language, affect, and behavior. Some of our recent research along these lines is summarized here.

8.1. Event-Related Potentials

Williamson et al. (1991) recorded reaction times and event-related potentials (ERPs) in a lexical decision task that required offenders to press a button as quickly and accurately as possible if a letter-string formed a word. The letter-strings were presented briefly on a computer screen, and consisted of neutral and emotional words and pronounceable pseudowords. Lexical decision studies with noncriminals indicate that responses to both positive words and negative words are more accurate and faster than are those to neutral words. Further, over central and parietal sites the early and late components of the ERP are larger in response to affective words than to neutral words. Increases in the amplitude of the early ERP components have been interpreted as a reflection of enhanced attentional processing of emotional words (e.g., Mangun, 1995), while increases in the amplitude of the late components are thought to be indicative of enhanced elaborative processing of emotional words (Rugg, 1985).

We found that, like noncriminals, nonpsychopathic criminals were sensitive to the affective manipulations of the lexical decision task. They responded faster to emotional words than to neutral words, and showed the expected ERP differentiation between the two word types. Psychopaths, on the other hand, failed to show any reaction time or ERP differences between neutral and emotional words. Further, the morphology of their ERPs was strikingly different from that of the nonpsychopaths. The late components were relatively small and brief in psychopaths, perhaps because they processed the information in a cursory, shallow manner and did little more than make a lexical decision, whereas the nonpsychopaths continued to process and mentally activate or *"elaborate"* the semantic and affective associations or networks of the word they had just seen. We also found another striking difference between psychopaths and nonpsychopaths. The psychopaths exhibited a very large negative-going wave (referred to as N500), most prominent over fronto-central cortex (Fz, Cz). In attempting to interpret this odd finding, we relied on evidence that similar negative components in normal individuals may reflect elaborative processes that serve to integrate the various attributes of a word, such as its meaning, into a context. We speculated that the large N500 in the psychopaths was related to difficulty in "integrating word meanings either within larger linguistic structures or with other conceptual structures" (Williamson et al, 1991, p. 269). Overall, the results of this study indicated that psychopaths show no behavioral or ERP differentiation between neutral and emotional words, and that they may have difficulty in placing words into an appropriate cognitive structure. If so, this would imply that psychopaths have serious linguistic problems.

A similar interpretation might be offered for the results of a study by Kiehl et al. (1999). We found that, unlike nonpsychopaths, psychopaths showed little or no ERP differentiation between negative and positive emotional words, or between concrete and abstract words. In each type of task, the psychopaths showed an unusually large fronto-central negative wave (referred to as N350).

We recently used ERPs and a Go/No Go task to investigate response inhibition in psychopathic, schizophrenic, and other (nonpsychotic, nonpsychopathic) offenders (Kiehl, Smith, Hare, & Liddle, 2000). The latter showed greater frontal ERP negativity (N275) to the No Go stimuli than to the Go stimuli. This difference between the No Go and Go stimuli was relatively small in schizophrenic offenders, and absent in psychopathic offenders. The neural generators of the N275 have not been localized precisely, but recent evidence from neuroimaging studies indicates that the anterior cingulated, lateral frontal cortex, and left superior frontal cortex may be involved in response inhibition (Carter, Braver, Barch, Botvinick, Noll, & Cohen, 1998; Kiehl, Liddle, & Hopfinger, 2000; Konishi et al, 1999). With respect to psychopathy, it is possible that our ERP results reflect anomalies in the neural sites or circuits related to response inhibition.

8.2. Single Photon Computed Tomography (SPECT)

Recently we conducted a SPECT study of relative cerebral blood flow (rCBF) in a lexical decision task performed by psychopathic substance abusers (Hare, 1998; Intrator et al, 1997). The premise of the study was that in normal subjects the cognitive demands imposed by a lexical decision task are associated with increases in activity in several parts of the brain, including prefrontal and temporal cortex. However, the results of the Williamson et al. study (1991) suggested that psychopaths generate relatively few semantic/affective associations during lexical decisions, and we therefore expected that they would show less widespread activation than would normal subjects. Each subject was presented with a block of neutral words and nonwords in one session, and a block of emotional (negative) words and nonwords in a separate session. The task was to press a button whenever a word appeared on the computer screen. We focused our attention on a mid-ventricular slice that encompassed prefrontal, anterior temporal, posterior temporal, temporal-parietal, and occipital cortex, as well as the basal ganglia and medial aspects of the frontal lobes. As described by Hare (1998), cortical activation in the psychopaths was far less widespread than it was in the other subjects. For the latter, there was activation in left hemisphere language areas and left thalamus during processing of the neutral words, and activation of right anterior areas during processing of emotional words, a pattern of activation that is appropriate given the nature of the tasks.

For psychopaths, however, the greatest activation was in occipital cortex, with considerably less activation in frontal, temporal, and parietal areas, particularly when they performed the neutral portion of the task. Of course, stimulus input for the task was visual and therefore initial processing occurred in occipital cortex, but the nonpsychopaths also did a lot of additional processing in more anterior regions of the brain, whereas the psychopaths did not engage in very much anterior processing, not even in language areas. Although it may be tempting to conclude that the psychopaths were not fully engaged in the task, perhaps because of drowsiness or boredom, there were no significant group differences in performance of the lexical decision task or in the speed-accuracy tradeoff. It is unlikely, therefore, that the SPECT results were related to group differences in level of alertness or motivation, at least to the extent that these factors are related to task performance. Similarly, all subjects had been screened for potentially confounding neurological, medical, and psychiatric disorders, suggesting that the relative lack of frontal activation in the psychopaths was not the result of palpable brain damage. However, the psychopaths differed less from the other patient group than from the comparison group, suggesting that at least part of the pattern of activation of the psychopaths was related to substance abuse.

This study also produced a curious finding. Psychopaths showed greater relative activation in the emotional than in the neutral condition, whereas the two non-psychopathic groups showed just the opposite pattern. These results surprised us, but they made (after the fact) sense, given evidence that metabolic demands (and rCBF) decrease as the cognitive operations associated with performance of a task become deeply embedded or overlearned (Gur, 1992). In many tasks, including linguistic ones of the sort used in the present study, these operations include efficient (automatic?) extraction and use of affective information. The ability to evaluate things as good or bad, as safe or dangerous, clearly has implications for our survival and well-being. This obviously requires the integration of several cognitive and affective processes. With respect to linguistic stimuli, for example, the individual presumably must determine the physical characteristics of the word, match this information with a stored (and retrieved) lexicon, extract and use the word's denotative and connotative/affective meanings, integrate these meanings with other percepts and stored experiences, and prepare to make a motor response. Several areas of the brain appear to be actively involved in the process, including extrastriate cortex, anterior regions responsible for semantic processing and response preparation, and –most important for our purposes– medial frontal-temporal regions that have strong afferent and efferent connections to the amygdala and that play an important role in elaborating the emotional significance of the stimulus (Damasio, 1994). In normal individuals the neurophysiological processes involved in decoding the affective information contained in words no doubt are so overlearned and efficient that metabolic requirements are minimal.

Psychopaths, on the other hand, seem to have difficulty in fully understanding and using words that for normal people refer to ordinary emotional events and feelings. Instead, they process and use them primarily in terms of denotative, dictionary meanings. It is as if emotion is a second language for psychopaths, a language that requires a considerable amount of mental transformation and cognitive effort on their part. It is possible that lexical decisions involving emotional words placed heavy demands on the psychopaths, and that the cortical and subcortical regions ordinarily involved in adding affect to language were very active (as reflected in increased rCBF) but relatively inefficient (Squire, 1987). This interpretation of our SPECT results is supported by the results of a recent functional magnetic imaging (fMRI) study by Schneider et al. (2000), described in the next section.

8.3. Functional Magnetic Resonance Imaging (fMRI)

Several recent fMRI studies by a team at my university are beginning to provide some interesting new clues on the neurobiological correlates of psychopathy. The framework for this research is the compelling evidence of the crucial roles played by ventromedial and dorsolateral frontal cortex in the integration and regulation of cognition, affect, and response inhibition. Because these studies are still in progress, only a few preliminary results are presented here.

In one study (Kiehl et al, 2001) subjects memorized a list of neutral and emotional words. Later, this list was embedded in a larger list, and the subjects were asked to identify the words that had appeared in the first list. We computed the difference in cortical activity between the neutral and emotional words for psychopaths and nonpsychopaths. Nonpsychopaths showed greater activation during processing of emotional words than did psychopaths in several limbic regions, including the amygdala, intimately involved in emotion, and the anterior and posterior cingulate, involved in emotional and attentional processes. These areas have rich connections with ventromedial frontal cortex. The importance of these regions for understanding psychopathy is clear. As Damasio (1994) put it, "One might say, metaphorically, that reason and emotion 'intersect' in the ventromedial frontal cortices, and that they also intersect in the amygdala... I would like to propose that there is a particular region in the human brain where the systems concerned with emotion/feeling, attention, and working memory intersect so intimately that they constitute the energy source of both external action (movement) and internal action (thought, animation, reasoning). This fountainhead region is the anterior cingulate cortex, another piece of the limbic system" (p. 70-71). The failure of ventromedial frontal cortex and associated limbic mechanisms to function properly would help to account for the apparent inability of psychopaths to experience deep-seated emotions and to process emotional material efficiently.

In another fMRI study (Smith, Hare, Kiehl, & Liddle, 2001) we used a Go/No Go task to investigate response inhibition in psychopathic and nonpsychopathic offenders. Like the ERP study of response inhibition (Kiehl et al, 2000), described above, psychopaths showed anomalies in activation in frontal regions, in this case, dorsolateral frontal cortex. In interpreting the results of these fMRI studies, we recognize that no regions of the brain operate independently, and that response inhibition must involve active integration and cooperation of many regions, including ventromedial and dorsolateral frontal cortex. In this regard, Pandya and Yeterian (1996) have suggested that the bi-directional intrinsic connections of ventromedial prefrontal cortex with lateral regions contribute in various ways to the process of decision making. For example, they influence response modulation, planning and sequencing of behavior, and attentional processes. They propose that the execution of appropriate responses, and the inhibition of inappropriate responses under changing circumstances are controlled by a combination of activities in ventromedial and dorsolateral prefrontal regions. The former serves functions that are crucial for the adaptability of behavior for survival, including the emotional and motivational formulation of decisions, and the latter provides further elaboration with regard to decision-making and to the actions that result from the decision.

Presumably, the disinhibitory behavior of psychopaths, including the ease with which they engage in predatory violence, is associated with functionally inadequate activity in ventromedial frontal cortex (cognitive/affective integration) *and* dorsolateral frontal cortex (response inhibition), and/or with ineffective communications among these and other regions of the brain (Smith, 1999). That is, the cortical/cognitive processes that ordinarily help to inhibit behavior are facilitated by intense emotional coloring in most people, but not in psychopaths. For them, the emotional "brakes" on behavior ("conscience?") are weak, allowing them to engage in predatory, violent acts without compunction. The problem may lie in underactivation of limbic regions, especially the amygdala and its neural connections (Blair & Cipolotti, 2000; Blair, Morris, Frith, Perret, & Dolan, 2000; Kiehl et al, 2001). However, the results of the SPECT study by Intrator et al. (1997), described above, suggested that it is also possible that these regions are not so much underactivated as they are ineffectively connected to cortical regions. Support for this possibility comes from a recent fMRI differential classical conditioning study of German forensic psychiatric patients with high PCL-R scores (Schneider et al., 2000). Two conditioned stimuli (pictures of a neutral face) were used, one (CS+)

followed by a puff of a noxious odor, the other (CS-) followed by a puff of odorless air. In healthy control subjects, the CS+ was associated with differential *decreases* (relative to the CS-) in activity in amygdala and dorsolateral prefrontal cortex, whereas the psychopaths showed *increases* in activation of these regions. One interpretation offered for these unexpected results was that the tasks placed relatively heavy processing demands on the psychopaths, an interpretation that "is consistent with a recent SPECT study (by Intrator et al, 1997) that demonstrated increased blood flow in subcortical regions of psychopaths during the processing of emotional words" (p. 199).

As a final point, I might note that at least some of these putative neurobiological anomalies could be related to abnormal neurotransmitter functions. If so, the apparently intractable behavior of psychopaths and their resistance to traditional treatment strategies (Wong & Hare, in press) might be responsive to biological interventions, particularly if introduced at an early age.

REFERENCES

American Psychiatric Association (1994): *Diagnostic and statistical manual of mental disorders* (4th ed.), Washington DC, Author.

Babiak, P. (1995): "When psychopaths go to work", *International Journal of Applied Psychology*, 44, pp. 171-188.

Barbaree, H.; Seto, M.; Serin, R.; Amos, N. & Preston, D. (1994): "Comparisons between sexual and nonsexual rapist subtypes", *Criminal Justice and Behavior,* 21, pp. 95-114.

Berrios, G. E. (1996*). The history of mental symptoms: Descriptive psychopathology since the nineteenth century*, Cambridge, Cambridge University Press.

Blair, R. J. R. & Cipolotti, L. (2000): "Impaired social reversal: A case of 'acquired' sociopathy", *Brain*, 123, pp. 1122-1141.

Blair, R. J. R.; Morris, J. S.; Frith, C. D.; Perret, D. I. & Dolan, R. J. (2000): "Dissociable neural responses to facial expressions of sadness and anger", *Brain*, 122, pp. 883-893.

Brandt, J. R.; Kennedy, W. A.; Patrick, C. J. & Curtin, J. J. (1997): "Assessment of psychopathy in a population of incarcerated adolescent offenders", *Psychological Assessment,* 9, pp. 429-435.

Brown, S. L. & Forth, A. E. (1997): "Psychopathy and sexual assault: Static risk factors, emotional precursors, and rapist subtypes", *Journal of Consulting and Clinical Psychology*, 65, pp. 848-857.

Carter, C. S.; Braver, T. S.; Barch, D. M.; Botvinick, M. M.; Noll, D. & Cohen, J. D. (1998): "Anterior cingulated cortex, error detection, and the online monitoring of performance", *Science*, 280, pp. 747-749.

Cleckley, H. (1976): *The mask of sanity* (5th ed.), St. Louis MO, Mosby.

Cooke, D. J.; Forth, A. E. & Hare, R. D. (eds.) (1998): *Psychopathy: Theory, research, and implications for society*, Dordrecht, The Netherlands, Kluwer.

Cooke, D. J. & Michie, C. (1997): "An Item Response Theory analysis of the Hare Psychopathy Checklist", *Psychological Assessment*, 9, pp. 3-13.

Cooke, D. J. & Michie, C. (1999): "Psychopathy across cultures: North America and Scotland compared", *Journal of Abnormal Psychology*, 108, pp.58-68.

Cooke , D. J. & Michie, C. (in press): "A hierarchical model of psychopathy: Replication and implications for measurement", *Psychological Assessment*.

Cooke, D. J.; Michie, C.; Hart, S. D. & Hare, R. D. (1999): "Evaluation of the screening version of the Hare Psychopathy Checklist-Revised (PCL:SV): An item response theory analysis", *Psychological Assessment*, 11, pp. 3-13.

Cornell, D. G.; Warren, J.; Hawk, G.; Stafford, E.; Oram, G. & Pine, D. (1996): "Psychopathy of instrumental and reactive violent offenders", *Journal of Consulting and Clinical Psychology*, 64, pp. 783-790.

Damasio, A. (1994): *Descartes' error: Emotion, reason, and the human brain*, New York, Putnam.

Dolan, B. & Coid, J. (1993): *Psychopathic and antisocial personality disorders: Treatment and research issues*, London, Gaskell.

Dolan, M. & Doyle, M. (2000): "Violence risk prediction: Clinical and actuarial measures and the role of the Psychopathy Checklist", *British Journal of Psychiatry*, 177, pp. 303-311.

Douglas, K. S.; Ogloff, J. R. P. & Nicholls, T. L. (1997, junio): *Personality disorders and violence in civil psychiatric patients*, Paper presented at the 5th International Congress on the Disorders of Personality, Vancouver, British Columbia.

Dutton, D. G. & Kropp, P. R. (2000): "A review of domestic violence risk instruments", *Trauma, Violence & Abuse*, 1, pp. 171- 181.

Edens, J. F.; Skeem, J. L.; Cruise, K. R. & Cauffman, E. (2001): "Assessment of "juvenile psychopathy" and its association with violence: A critical review", *Behavioral Sciences and the Law*, 19, pp. 53-80.

Federal Bureau of Investigation (1992): *Killed in the line of duty*, Washington DC, United States Department of Justice.

Firestone, P.; Bradford, J. M.; Greenberg, D. M. & Larose, M. R. (1998): "Homicidal sex offenders: Psychological, phallometric, and diagnostic features", *Journal of the American Academy of Psychiatry and Law*, 26, pp. 537-552.

Forth, A. E., (1995): *Psychopathy and young offenders: Prevalence, family background, and violence*, Programs Branch Users Report, Ottawa - Ontario, Ministry of the Solicitor General of Canada.

Forth, A. E.; Brown, S. L.; Hart, S. D. & Hare, R. D. (1996): "The assessment of psychopathy in male and female noncriminals: Reliability and validity", *Personality and Individual Differences*, 20, pp. 531-543.

Forth, A. E. & Burke, H. (1998): "Psychopathy in adolescence: Assessment, violence, and developmental precursors", in R. D. Cooke, A. E. Forth & R. D. Hare (eds.), *Psychopathy: Theory, research, and implications for society*, Dordrecht, The Netherlands, Kluwer, pp. 205-229.

Forth, A. E.; Hart, S. D. & Hare, R. D. (1990): "Assessment of psychopathy in male young offenders", *Psychological Assessment*, 2, pp. 342-344.

Forth, A. E.; Kosson, D. & Hare, R. D. (in press): *The Hare Psychopathy Checklist: Youth Version*, Toronto-Ontario, Multi-Health Systems.

Frick, P.J. (1998): "Callous-emotional traits and conduct problems: Applying the two-factor model of psychopathy to children", in D. J. Cooke, A. E. Forth & R. D. Hare (eds.): *Psychopathy: Theory, research, and implications for society*, Dordrecht, The Netherlands, Kluwer.

Fulero, S. M. (1995): "Review of the Hare Psychopathy Checklist-Revised", in J. C. Conoley & J. C. Impara (eds.), *Twelfth mental measurements yearbook*, Lincoln NE, Buros Institute., pp. 453-454.

Fuster, J. M. (1997): *The prefrontal cortex: Anatomy, physiology and neuropsychology of the frontal lobe* (3[a] ed.), Philadelphia PA, Lippincott-Raven.

Gillstrom, B. (1995): *Abstract thinking in criminal Psychopaths*, Unpublished doctoral dissertation, University of British Columbia, Vancouver, Canada.

Gorenstein, E. E. & Newman, J. P. (1980): "Disinhibitory psychopathology: A new perspective and a model for research", *Psychological Review*, 87, pp. 301-315.

Grann, M.; Langström, N.; Tengström, A. & Kullgren, G. (1999): "Psychopathy (PCL-R) predicts violent recidivism among criminal offenders with personality disorders in Sweden", *Law and Human Behavior,* 23, pp. 205-217.

Gretton, H. M. (1998): *Psychopathy and recidivism in adolescence: A ten-year retrospective follow-up*, Unpublished doctoral dissertation, University of British Columbia, Vancouver, Canada.

Gretton, H. M.; McBride, M.; Hare, R. D.; O'Shaughnessy, R. & Kumka, G. (in press): "Psychopathy and recidivism in adolescent sex offenders", *Criminal Justice and Behavior.*

Grisolía, J. S.; Sanmartin, J.; Luján, J. L. & Grisolía, S. (eds.) (1997): *Violence: from biology to society*, Amsterdam, Elsevier.

Gustaffson, S. B. & Ritzer, D. R. (1995): "The dark side of normal: A Psychopathy-linked pattern called aberrant self-promotion", *European Journal of Personality, 9*, pp. 1-37.

Hare, R. D. (1985): "A comparison of procedures for the assessment of psychopathy", *Journal of Consulting and Clinical Psychology*, 53, pp. 7-16.

Hare, R. D. (1991): *The Hare Psychopathy Checklist-Revised*, Toronto, Canada, Multi-Health Systems.

Hare, R. D. (1993): *Without conscience: The disturbing world of the psychopaths among us*, New York, Pocket Books. Reissued in 1998 by Guilford Press.

Hare, R. D. (1998): "Psychopathy, affect, and behavior", in D. J. Cooke, A. E. Forth & R. D. Hare (eds.), *Psychopathy: Theory, research, and implications for society*, Dordrecht, The Netherlands, Kluwer.

Hare, R. D. (1999): "Psychopathy as a risk factor for violence", *Psychiatric Quarterly,* 70, pp. 181-197.

Hare, R. D.; Clark, D.; Grann, M. & Thornton, D. (2000). "Psychopathy and the predictive validity of the PCL-R: An international perspective", *Behavioral Sciences and the Law*, 18, pp. 623-645.

Hare, R. D. & Hart, S. D. (1995): "A commentary on the Antisocial Personality Disorder Field Trial", in W. J. Livesley (ed.), *The DSM-IV personality disorders*, New York, Guilford.

Hare, R. D.; McPherson, L. E. & Forth, A. E. (1988): "Male psychopaths and their criminal careers", *Journal of Consulting and Clinical Psychology*, 56, pp. 710-714.

Harpur, T. J. & Hare, R. D. (1994): "The assessment of psychopathy as a function of age", *Journal of Abnormal Psychology*, 103, pp. 604-609.

Harris, A. J. R. & Hanson, R. K. (1998, October): *Supervising the psychopathic sex deviant in the community*, Paper presented at the 17th Annual Research and Treatment Conference, The Association for the Treatment of Sexual Abusers, Vancouver, Canada.

Harris, G. T.; Rice, M. E. & Cormier, C. A. (1991): "Psychopathy and violent recidivism", *Law and Human Behavior, 15*, pp. 625-637.

Harris, G. T.; Rice, M. E. & Quinsey, V. L. (1993): "Violent recidivism of mentally disordered offenders: The development of a statistical prediction instrument", *Criminal Justice and Behavior*, 20, pp. 315-335.

Hart, S. D.; Cox, D. N. & Hare, R. D. (1995): *The Hare Psychopathy Checklist: Screening Version*, Toronto, Canada, Multi-Health Systems.

Hart, S. D.; Forth, A. E. & Hare, R. D. (1990): "Neuropsychological assessment of criminal psychopaths", *Journal of Abnormal Psychology*, 99, pp. 374-379.

Hart, S. D. & Hare, R. D. (1989): "Discriminant validity of the Psychopathy Checklist in a forensic psychiatric population", *Psychological Assessment*, 1, pp. 211-218.

Hart, S. D. & Hare, R. D. (1997): "Psychopathy: Assessment and association with criminal conduct", in D. M. Stoff, J. Brieling & J. Maser (eds.), *Handbook of antisocial behavior*, New York, Wiley, (pp. 22-35).

Hart, S. D.; Kropp, P. R. & Hare, R. D. (1988): "Performance of psychopaths following conditional release from prison", *Journal of Consulting and Clinical Psychology*, 56, pp. 227-232.

Heilbrun, K.; Hart, S. D.; Hare, R. D.; Gustafson, D.; Nunez, C. & White, A. (1998): "Inpatient and post-discharge aggression in mentally disordered offenders: The role of psychopathy", *Journal of Interpersonal Violence*, 13, pp. 514-527.

Hemphill, J. (1991): *Psychopathy and recidivism following release from a therapeutic community treatment program*, Unpublished master's thesis, University of Saskatchewan, Saskatoon, Saskatchewan, Canada.

Hemphill, J. F.; Hare, R. D. & Wong, S. (1998): "Psychopathy and recidivism: A review", *Legal and Criminological Psychology,* 3, pp. 141-172.

Hemphill, J.; Hart, S. D. & Hare, R. D. (1994): "Psychopathy and substance use", *Journal of Personality Disorders, 8,* pp. 32-40.

Hemphill, J. F.; Strachan, C. & Hare, R. D. (1999): *Psychopathy in female offenders*, Manuscript in preparation.

Hill, C. D.; Rogers, R. & Bickford, M. E. (1996): "Predicting aggressive and socially disruptive behavior in a maximum security forensic psychiatric hospital", *Journal of Forensic Sciences*, 41, pp. 56-59.

Hobson, J.; Shine, J. & Roberts, R. (2000): "How do psychopaths behave in a prison therapeutic prison community?", *Crime, and Law Psychology*, 6, pp. 139-154.

Huss, M. T. & Langhinrischen-Rohling, J. (2000): "Identification of the psychopathic batterer: The clinical, legal, and policy implications", *Aggression and Violent Behavior*, 5, pp. 403-422.

Intrator, J.; Hare, R.; Strizke, P.; Brichtswein, K.; Dorfman, D.; Harpur, T.; Bernstein, D.; Handelsman, L.; Schaefer, C.; Keilp, J.; Rosen, J. & Machac, J. (1997): "Brain imaging (SPECT) study of semantic and affective processing in Psychopaths", *Biological Psychiatry, 42*, pp. 96-103.

Kiehl, K. A.; Hare, R. D.; McDonald, J. J. & Brink, J. (1999): "Semantic and affective processing in psychopaths: An event-related potential (ERP) study", *Psychophysiology*., 36, pp. 765-774.

Kiehl, K. A.; Liddle, P. F. & Hopfinger, J. B. (2000): "Error processing in the rostral anterior cingulated: An event-related fMRIIII study", *Psychophysiology*, 37, pp. 216-223.

Kiehl, K. A.; Smith, A. M.; Hare, R. D. & Liddle, P. F. (2000): "An event-related potential investigation of response inhibition in schizophrenia and psychopathy", *Biological Psychiatry*, 48, pp. 210-221.

Kiehl, K. A.; Smith, A. M.; Mendrek, A.; Forster, B. B.; Hare, R. D. & Liddle, P. F. (2001): *Reduced limbic activity in criminal psychopaths during an affective memory task*, manuscript in preparation.

Konishi, S.; Naaaakajima, K.; Uchida, I.; Kikyo, H.; Kameyama, M. & Miyashita, Y. (1999): "Common inhibitory mechanism in human inferior prefrontal cortex revealed by event-related functional MRI", *Brain*, 122, pp. 981-991.

Kosson, D. S. & Harpur, T. J. (1997): "Attentional functioning of psychopathic individuals: Current evidence and developmental implications", in J. A. Burack & J. T. Enns (eds.), *Attention: Development and psychopathology*, New York, Guilford Press, pp. 379-402.

Lapierre, D.; Braun, C. M. J. & Hodgins, S. (1995): "Ventral frontal deficits in psychopathy: Neuropsychological test findings", *Neuropsychologia*, 33, pp. 139-151.

Liddle, P. F.; Smith, A. M.; Kiehl, K. A.; Mendrek, A. & Hare, R. D. (1999, April): *Response inhibition in schizophrenia and psychopathy: Similarities and differences*, Paper presented at the International Congress of Schizophrenia Research, Santa Fe, California.

Livesley, W. J. (1998): "The phenotypic and genotypic structure of psychopathic traits", in D. J. Cooke, A. E. Forth & R. D. Hare (eds.), *Psychopathy: Theory, research, and implications for society*, Dordrecht, The Netherlands, Kluwer.

Lösel, F. (1998): "Treatment and management of psychopaths", in D. J. Cooke, A. E. Forth & R. D. Hare (eds.), *Psychopathy: Theory, research, and implications for society*, Dordrecht, The Netherlands, Kluwer.

Lykken, D. T. (1995): *The antisocial personalities*, Hillsdale NJ, Erlbaum.

Lynam, D. R. (1996): "Early identification of chronic offenders: Who is the fledgling psychopath?", *Psychological Bulletin*, 120, pp. 209-234.

McBride, M. (1998): *Individual and familial risk factors for adolescent psychopathy*. Unpublished doctoral dissertation, University of British Columbia, Vancouver, Canada.

McCord, W. & McCord, J. (1964): *The psychopath: An essay on the criminal mind*, Princeton NJ, Van Nostrand.

Mealey, L. (1995): "The sociobiology of sociopathy: An integrated evolutionary model", *Behavioral and Brain Sciences*, 18, pp. 523-599.

Miller, M. W.; Geddings, V. J.; Levenston, G. K. & Patrick, C. J. (1994, marzo): *The personality characteristics of psychopathic and nonpsychopathic sex offenders*, Paper presented at the Reunión Bianual de la American Psychology-Law Society (Div. 41 of the American Psychological Association), Santa Fe, New Mexico.

Millon, T.; Simonsen, E.; Birket-Smith, M. & Davis, R. D. (1998): *Psychopathy: Antisocial, criminal, and violent behaviors*, New York, Guilford Press.

Murphy, J. M. (1976): "Psychiatric labelling in cross-cultural perspective: Similar kinds of disturbed behavior appear to be labelled abnormal in diverse cultures", *Science*, 191, pp. 1019-1028.

Newman, J. P. (1998): "Psychopathic behavior: An information processing perspective", in D. J. Cooke, A. E. Forth & R. D. Hare (eds.), *Psychopathy: Theory, research, and implications for society*, Dordrecht, The Netherlands, Kluwer.

Ogloff, J.; Wong, S. & Greenwood, A. (1990): "Treating criminal psychopaths in a therapeutic community program", *Behavioral Sciences and the Law*, 8, pp. 81-90.

Patrick, C. J. (1994): "Emotion and psychopathy: Some startling new insights", *Psychophysiology*, 31, pp. 319-330.

Pichot, P. (1978): "Psychopathic behavior: A historical overview", in R. D. Hare & D. Schalling (eds.), *Psychopathic behavior: Approaches to research*, Chichester UK, John Wiley, pp. 55-70.Porter, S.; Fairweather, D.; Drugge, J.; Hervé, H.; Birt, A. & Boer, D. P. (2000): "Profiles of psychopathy in incarcerated sexual offenders", *Criminal Justice and Behavior*, 27, pp. 216-233.

Quinsey, V. L.; Harris, G. E.; Rice, M. E. & Lalumiere, M. L. (1993): "Assessing treatment efficacy in outcome studies of sex offenders", *Journal of Interpersonal Violence*, 8, pp. 512-523.

Quinsey, V. L.; Rice, M. E. & Harris, G. T. (1995): "Actuarial prediction of sexual recidivism", *Journal of Interpersonal Violence,* 10, pp. 85-105.

Rice, M. E. & Harris, G. T. (1992): "A comparison of criminal recidivism among schizophrenic and nonschizophrenic offenders", *International Journal of Law and Psychiatry*, 15, pp. 397-408.

Rice, M. E. & Harris, G. T. (1997): "Cross-validation and extension of the Violence Risk Appraisal Guide for child molesters and rapists", *Law and Human Behavior*, 21, pp. 231-241.

Rice, M. E.; Harris, G. T. & Cormier, C. A. (1992): "An evaluation of a maximum security therapeutic community for psychopaths and other mentally disordered offenders", *Law and Human Behavior*, 16, pp. 399-412.

Robins, L. N. (1978): "Aetiological implications in studies of childhood histories relating to antisocial personality", in R. D. Hare & D. Schalling (eds.), *Psychopathic behavior: Approaches to research*, Chichester UK, John Wiley, pp. 255-271.

Salekin, R.; Rogers, R. & Sewell, K. (1996): "A review and meta-analysis of the Psychopathy Checklist and Psychopathy Checklist-Revised: Predictive validity of dangerousness", *Clinical Psychology: Science and Practice,* 3, pp. 203-215.

Salekin, R.; Rogers, R. & Sewell, K. (1997): "Construct validity of psychopathy in a female offender sample: A multitrait-multimethod evaluation", *Journal of Abnormal Psychology*, 106, pp. 576-585.

Salekin, R.W.; Rogers, R.; Ustad, K.L. & Sewell, K.W. (1998): "Psychopathy and recidivism among female inmates", *Law and Human Behavior, 22*, pp. 109-128.

Schneider, F.; Habel, U.; Kessler, C.; Posse, S.; Grodd, W. & Müller-Gartner, H. (2000): "Functional imaging of conditioned aversive emotional responses in antisocial personality disorder", *Neuropsychobiology*, 42, pp. 192-201.

Serin, R. C. & Amos, N. L. (1995): "The role of psychopathy in the assessment of dangerousness", *International Journal of Law and Psychiatry*, 18, pp. 231-238.

Serin, R. C.; Malcolm, P. B.; Khanna, A. & Barbaree, H. E. (1994): "Psychopathy and deviant sexual arousal in incarcerated sexual offenders", *Journal of Interpersonal Violence*, 9, pp. 3-11.

Silver, E.; Mulvey, E. P. & Monahan, J. (1999): "Assessing violence risk among discharged psychiatric patients: Toward an ecological approach", *Law and Human Behavior*, 23, pp. 237-255.

Squire, L. R. (1987): "Memory: Neural organization and behavior", in F. Plum (ed.), *Handbook of Physiology. The Nervous System*, Bethesda, MD, American Physiological Society.

Steadman, H. J.; Silver, E.; Monahan, J.; Appelbaum, P. S.; Robbins, P. M.; Mulvey, E. P.; Grisso, T.; Roth, L. H. & Banks, S. (2000): "A classification tree approach to the development of actuarial violence risk assessment tools", *Law and Human Behavior*, 24, pp. 83-100.

Stone, M. H. (1998): "The personalities of murderers: The importance of psychopathy and sadism", in A. E. Skodol (ed.), *Psychopathology and violent crime*, Washington DC, American Psychiatric Association, pp. 29-52.

Suedfeld, P. & Landon, P.B. (1978): "Approaches to treatment", in R. D. Hare & D. Schalling (eds.): *Psychopathic behavior: Approaches to research*, Chichester UK, Wiley, pp. 347-376.

Tengström, A.; Grann, M.; Langström, N. & Kullgren, G. (2000): "Psychopathy (PCL-R) as a predictor of violent recidivism among criminal offenders with schizophrenia", *Law and Human Behavior*, 24, pp. 45-58.

Toupin, J.; Mercier, H.; Dery, M.; Côté, G. & Hodgins, S. (1996): "Validity of the PCL-R for adolescents", in D. J. Cooke, A. E. Forth, J. P. Newman & R. D. Hare (eds.), *Issues in Criminological and Legal Psychology, No. 24*, *International perspectives on psychopathy*, Leicester UK, British Psychological Society, pp. 143-145.

Tucker, W. (1999): "The 'mad' vs. the 'bad' revisited: Managing predatory behavior", *Psychiatric Quarterly, 70, pp. 221-230*Widiger, T. A. (1998): "Psychopathy and normal personality", in D. J. Cooke, A. E. Forth & R. D. Hare (eds.), *Psychopathy: Theory, research, and implications for society*, Dordrecht, The Netherlands, Kluwer.

Widiger, T. A.; Cadoret, R.; Hare, R. D.; Robins, L.; Rutherford, M.; Zanarini, M.; Alterman, A.; Apple, M.; Corbitt, E.; Forth, A.; Hart, S.; Kulterman, J. & Woody, G. (1996): "DSM-IV Antisocial Personality Disorder Field Trial", *Journal of Abnormal Psychology*, 105, pp. 3-16.

Widiger, T. A. & Corbitt, E. (1995): "The DSM-IV Antisocial Personality Disorder", in W. J. Livesley (ed.), *The DSM-IV personality disorders*, New York, Guilford.

Williamson, S. E.; Harpur, T. J. & Hare, R. D. (1991): "Abnormal processing of affective words by psychopaths", *Psychophysiology,* 28, pp. 260-273.

Wilson, J. Q. & Herrnstein, R. J. (1985): *Crime and human nature*, New York, Simon & Schuster.

Wintrup, A. (1994): *The predictive validity of the PCL-R in high risk mentally disordered offenders*, Unpublished manuscript, Simon Fraser University, Burnaby, British Columbia, Canada.

Wong, S. & Hare, R. D. (in press): *Program guidelines for the institutional treatment of violent psychopaths*, Toronto, Canada, Multi-Health Systems.

World Health Organization (1990): *International classification of diseases and related health problems* (10th ed.), Genera, Switzerland, Author.

Chapter 2

PSYCHOPATHY, VIOLENCE, AND BRAIN IMAGING

Adrian Raine
Department of Psychology, University of Southern California, USA

1. INTRODUCTION: PREVIOUS BRAIN IMAGING STUDIES OF OFFENDERS

Advances in brain imaging techniques in the past 15 years have provided the opportunity to gain dramatic, new insights into the brain mechanisms that may be dysfunctional in violent, psychopathic offenders. In the past, the idea of peering into the mind of a murderer to gain insights into their acts was the province of pulp fiction or space-age movies. Yet now we can literally look at, and into, the brains of murderers using functional and structural imaging techniques which are currently revolutionizing our understanding of the causes of clinical disorders.

Brain imaging studies of violent and psychopathic offenders are particularly important because they offer a new paradigm to confirm, refute, or modify the conclusions which have been drawn from findings of prior neurological and neuropsychological studies. With respect to the cerebral cortex, such animal and human studies have implicated dysfunction to the frontal (Benson and Miller, 1997; Damasio, 1994) as well as the temporal regions of the brain (Grisolia, 1997). Subcortically, experimental studies have shown that the amygdala, hippocampus, hypothalamus, and periaqueductal gray are all involved in the generation and regulation of aggression (Grisolia, 1997; Mirsky and Siegel, 1994). The critical question, therefore, is whether imaging studies are beginning to substantiate findings from this older literature.

Brain imaging studies of violent and psychopathic populations have been reviewed by Raine (1993), Raine and Buchsbaum (1996), and Henry and Moffitt (1997). These reviews (which cover studies up to 1994), while showing variability in findings across studies, concur in indicating that violent offenders have structural and functional deficits to the anterior

Violence and Psychopathy, edited by Raine & Sanmartin,
Kluwer Academic/Plenum Publishers, New York, 2001.

regions of the brain, that is, the frontal lobe and the temporal lobe. There is a trend for temporal lobe abnormalities to be especially found in sex offenders (Henry and Moffitt, 1997; Raine, 1993), but this conclusion requires further elaboration and clarification.

Since these reviews, five more recent studies support this key finding of anterior brain dysfunction. Goyer et al. (1994) using positron emission tomography (PET) in an auditory activation condition showed that an increased number of aggressive impulsive acts were associated with reduced glucose in the frontal cortex of 17 personality-disordered patients. Volkow et al. (1995) using PET in a non-activation, eyes open, resting state observed reduced glucose metabolism in both prefrontal and medial temporal regions in 8 psychiatric patients (three with schizophrenia) with a history of violence. Kuruoglu et al. (1996) using single photon emission computerized tomography (SPECT) in a resting state found that 15 alcoholics with antisocial personality disorder showed significantly reduced frontal regional cerebral blood flow (rCBF) compared to 4 alcoholics with other personality disorders and 10 nonalcoholic controls. Seidenwurm et al. (1997) using PET in a non-activation, eyes open, resting state found a significant reduction in glucose metabolism in the medial temporal lobe in 7 violent offenders (2 schizophrenic) referred for forensic examination and suspected of organic brain disease. Intrator et al. (1997) using SPECT showed that 8 drug-abusing psychopaths compared to 9 non-psychopaths had increased rCBF bilaterally in fronto-temporal regions during the processing of emotional words.

Taken together, these later studies show continued support of the notion of poor functioning of the frontal and temporal regions of the brain in antisocial individuals, with poor frontal functioning being particularly salient. Out of the five studies, four showed evidence for frontal dysfunction while three showed evidence for temporal lobe dysfunction. Despite some discrepancies, the first generation of brain imaging studies support earlier contentions from animal and neurological studies implicating the frontal and temporal regions in the regulation and expression of aggression. A critical gap in the field to date, however, is the lack of findings on subcortical regions such as the amygdala and hippocampus.

With this literature as a background, the remainder of this paper explores in more detail the notion that prefrontal dysfunction may be an important predisposition to violent, antisocial, and psychopathic behavior with reference to new brain imaging studies. The central questions that will be addressed are (1) does prefrontal dysfunction characterize murderers? (2) what other cortical and subcortical brain structures are dysfunctional in this group (3) does prefrontal dysfunction characterize a subgroup of murderers who are impulsive and emotional? (4) how do psychosocial deficits moderate the link between brain dysfunction and violence? (5) can structural deficits to the prefrontal cortex be found in those with a diagnosis of antisocial personality disorder in the community? (6) do these deficits relate to psychopathic personality? (7) what are the mechanisms and processes through which prefrontal and autonomic deficits predispose to antisocial personality disorder? Answers to these question will then be followed with a discussion of the philosophical, moral, legal, and political issues posed by brain imaging research in offender populations.

2. PREFRONTAL DYSFUNCTION IN MURDERERS

Do prefrontal deficits characterize murderers? In the first published brain imaging study of murderers (Raine et al., 1994), we scanned the brains of 41 murderers pleading not-guilty by reason of insanity (or else incompetent to stand trial), and compared them to the brains of 41 normal controls who were matched with the murderers on sex and age. The technique we used was positron emission tomography which allowed us to measure the metabolic activity of many different regions of the brain, including the prefrontal cortex, the frontal-most part of the brain. We used the continuous performance task to "challenge" or activate the prefrontal cortex. This visual task requires the subject to maintain focused attention and be vigilant for a continuous period of time, and it is the prefrontal region of the brain that in part subserves this vigilance function.

The key finding of the study is illustrated in Figure 1 which shows the brain scan of a normal control (left) and the brain scan of a murderer (right) who impulsively killed his victim. The figure shows a transverse (horizontal) slice through the brain, so you are looking down on it with the prefrontal region at the top, and the occipital cortex (the back part of the brain controlling vision) at the bottom. Warm colors (e.g. red and yellow) indicate areas of high glucose metabolism, or high brain functioning, whereas cold colors (e.g. blue and green) indicate areas of low activation.

The striking difference between the two lies in the prefrontal cortex which is located at the top of Figure 1. The control subject on the left shows a lot of activation, while the murderer on the right shows very little activation. At the bottom of each scan it can be seen that the occipital cortex is activated about equally in both normal and murderer. This brain area which makes up the visual cortex is activated because the challenge task was visual. The deficit in the murderers was selective; no deficit was found in the temporal region, and as is indicated in Figure 1, the occipital cortex was at least as well activated in the murderer as in the control.

We think that poorer functioning of the prefrontal cortex predisposes to violence for a number of reasons. At a neurophysiological level, reduced prefrontal functioning can result in a loss of inhibition or control on phylogenetically older subcortical structures such as the amygdala, which

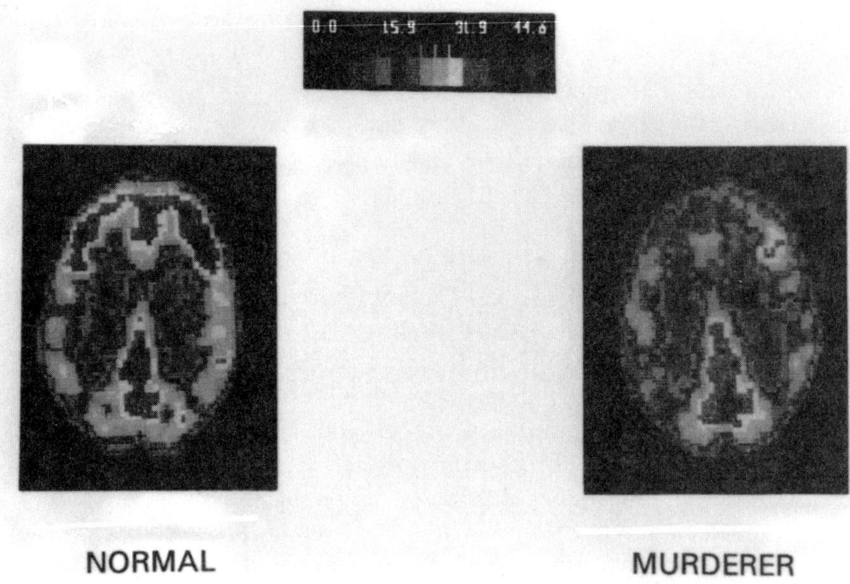

Figure 1. PET scan of normal control (left) and murderer (right) showing reduced activation in the prefrontal cortex of the murderer (upper part of figure). Color version of figure appears following page 38.

are thought to give rise to aggressive feelings. At a neurobehavioral level, prefrontal damage has been found to result in risk taking, irresponsibility, rule-breaking, emotional and aggressive outbursts, and argumentative behavior which can also predispose to violent criminal acts. At a personality level, frontal damage in neurological patients is associated with impulsivity, loss of self-control, immaturity, lack of tact, inability to modify and inhibit behavior appropriately, and poor social judgment which could predispose to violence. At a social level, the loss of intellectual flexibility, problem-solving skills, and reduced ability to use information provided by verbal cues resulting from prefrontal dysfunction can impair social skills essential for formulating nonaggressive solutions to fractious encounters. At a cognitive level, poor reasoning ability and divergent thinking which results from prefrontal damage can result in school failure, unemployment, and economic deprivation, thereby predisposing to a criminal and violent way of life. Nevertheless, it should be recognized that while there is an association between poor prefrontal function and violence, this brain dysfunction may be essentially a predisposition only, requiring other environmental, psychological and social factors to enhance or diminish this biological predisposition.

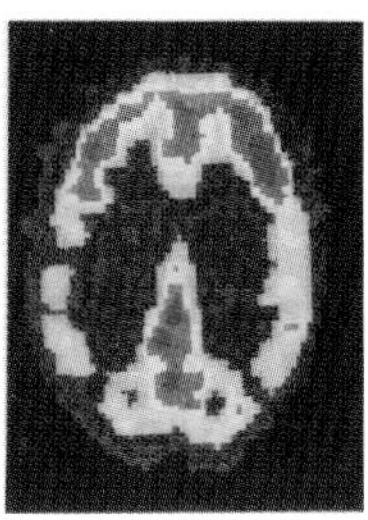

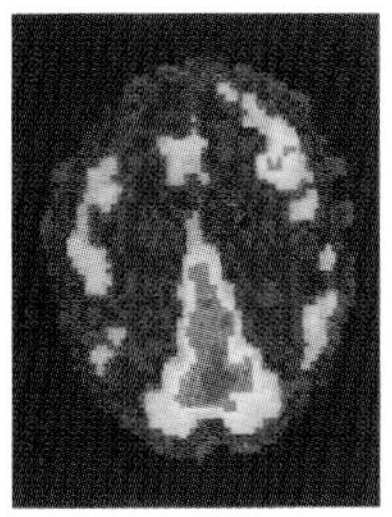

NORMAL **MURDERER**

Figure 1. PET scan of normal control (left) and murderer (right) showing reduced activation in the prefrontal cortex of the murderer (upper part of figure). Increased glucose metabolism is indicated by red and yellow while areas of low glucose metabolism are indicated by green and blue.

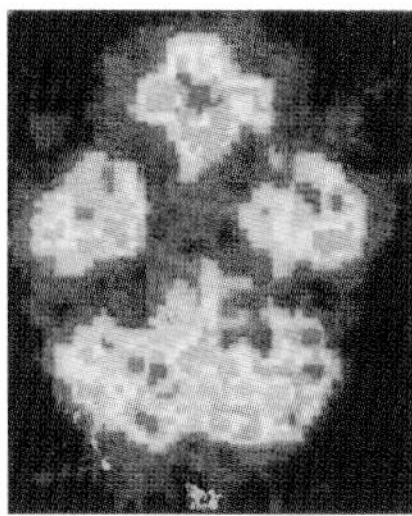

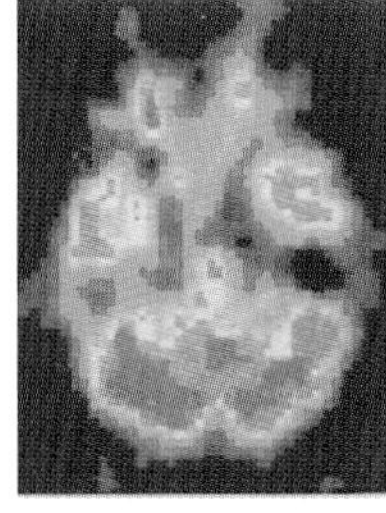

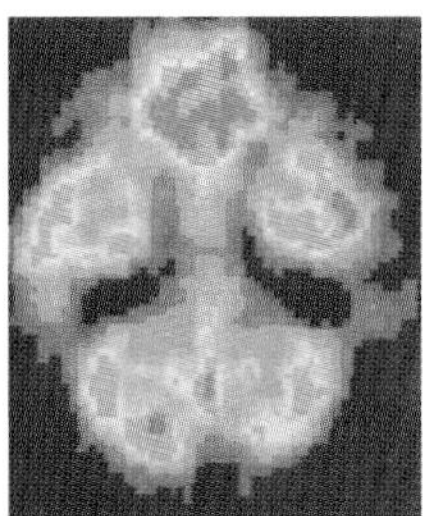

CONTROL AFFECTIVE PREDATORY

Figure 2. PET scan of normal control (left), affective murderer (middle), and predatory murderer (right) illustrating reduced prefrontal functioning in the affective murderer. Increased glucose metabolism is indicated by red and yellow while areas of low glucose metabolism are indicated by green and blue.

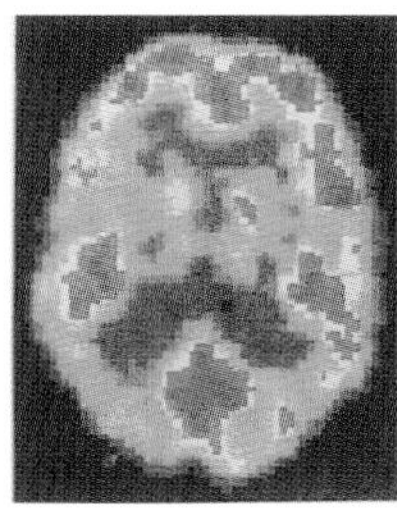

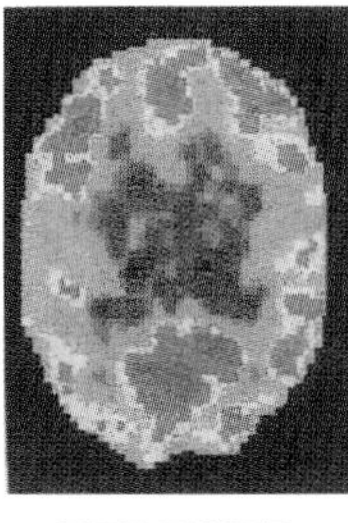

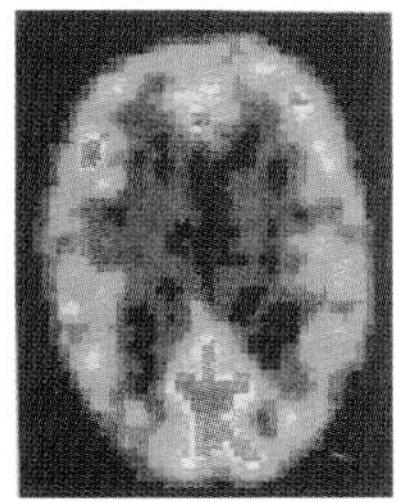

NORMAL CONTROL **DEPRIVED MURDERER** **NON-DEPRIVED MURDERER**

Figure 3. PET scan of normal control (left), murderer from deprived home background (middle) and murderer from benign home background (right) illustrating reduced prefrontal functioning in the non-socially deprived murderer. Increased glucose metabolism is indicated by red and yellow while areas of low glucose metabolism are indicated by green and blue.

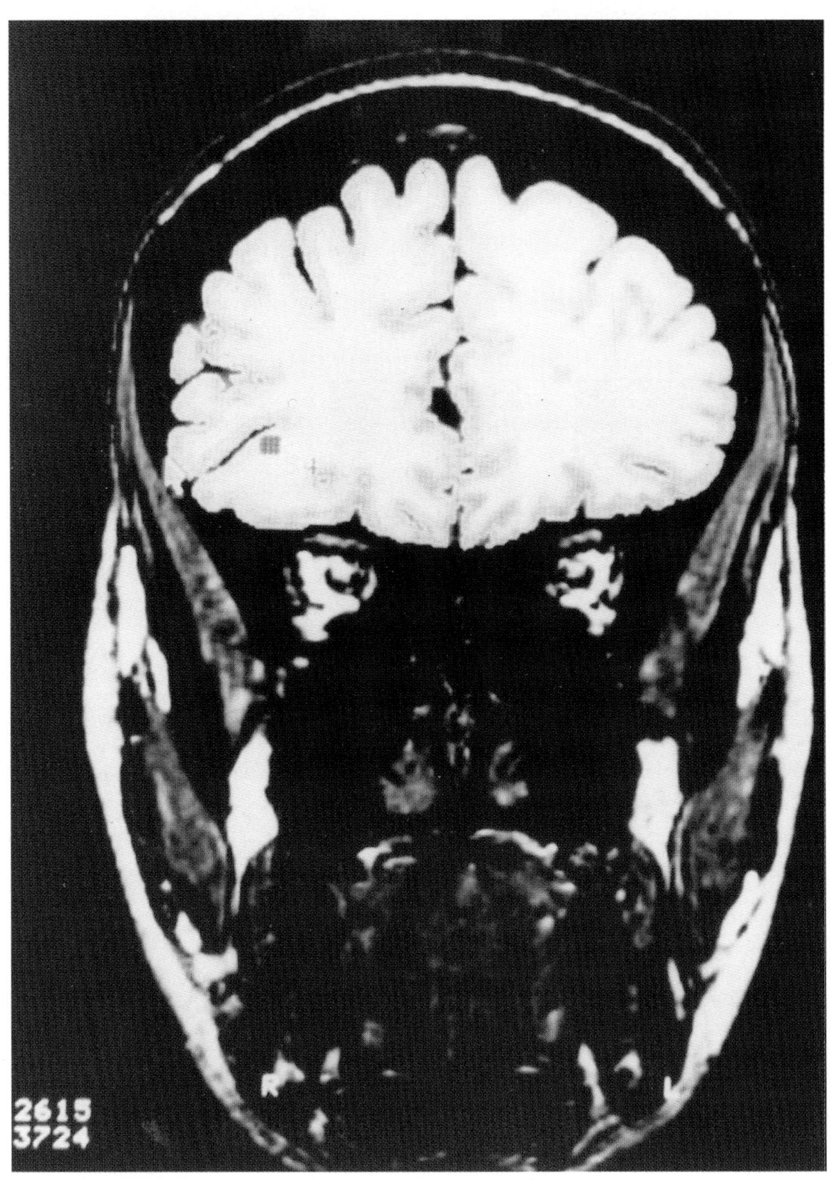

Figure 4. MRI coronal slice of the prefrontal cortex illustrating the seeding program for segmenting gray from white matter.

3. FURTHER FINDINGS: CORPUS CALLOSUM, LEFT ANGULAR GYRUS, AND THE SUBCORTEX

What other brain deficits, apart from prefrontal dysfunction, characterize murderers? We took this imaging research a step further by expanding our sample from 22 to 41 murderers, and also by increasing the size of our control group to 41. This increase in sample size gave us more statistical power to detect group differences, and in 1997 we reported our updated findings (Raine et al., 1997). The results were interesting for a variety of reasons. First, we confirmed that there was a significant reduction in the activity of the prefrontal region in murderers.

Second, we now found in this larger sample that the left angular gyrus was functioning more poorly in the murderers. The angular gyrus lies at the junction of the temporal, parietal, and occipital regions of the brain and plays a key role in integrating information from these three lobes. Reductions in glucose metabolism in the left angular gyrus have been correlated with reduced verbal ability (Gur et al., 1994), while damage to this region has been linked to deficits in reading and arithmetic. Such cognitive deficits could predispose to educational and occupational failure which in turn predisposes to crime and violence. The fact that learning deficits have been found to be common in violent offenders lends further support to this interpretation.

Third, we found reductions in the functioning of the corpus callosum, the band of white nerve fibers that provides lines of communication between the left and right hemispheres. Although we can only speculate at the present time, we think that poor connection between the hemispheres may mean that the right hemisphere, which is involved in the generation of negative emotion (Davidson and Fox, 1989) may experience less regulation and control by the inhibitory processes of the more dominant left hemisphere, a factor which may contribute to the expression of violence. Interestingly, rats stressed early in life are right hemisphere dominant for mouse killing (Garbanti et al., 1983). Severing the corpus callosum in these rats results in an increase in muricide (Denenberg et al., 1986), indicating that the left hemisphere normally acts to inhibit the right hemisphere's mouse-killing tendency. Furthermore, researchers have commented on the inappropriate nature of emotional expression and the inability to grasp long-term implications of a situation in split-brain patients who have had their corpus callosum surgically severed. This implies that the inappropriate emotional expression of violent offenders and their lack of long-term planning may be partly accounted for by poor functioning of the corpus callosum. Nevertheless, callosal dysfunction by itself is unlikely to cause aggression. Instead, it may only contribute to violence in those who also have other limbic and cortical abnormalities.

Fourth, we also observed unusual functioning in subcortical regions, including the amygdala, hippocampus, and thalamus. Murderers tended to show relatively greater lower left (but greater right) functioning in these structures. While the exact interpretations of these findings are currently speculative, it is no great surprise that these structures function abnormally in murderers. The amygdala has been repeatedly associated with aggressive behavior in both animals and humans (Mirsky and Siegel, 1994). It makes up part of the neural network that forms the basis to the processing of socially relevant information, and functions in parallel with the object recognition system of the hippocampus. Disruption to such a system could in part relate to the socially-inappropriate behavior shown by some violent individuals and the misrecognition and misappraisal of ambiguous stimuli in social situations which have potential for violent encounters (Dodge et al., 1990).

More generally, the amygdala, hippocampus, and prefrontal cortex make up part of the limbic system governing the expression of emotion, while the thalamus relays inputs from subcortical limbic structures to the prefrontal cortex (Fuster, 1989; Dodge et al., 1990). The hippocampus, amygdala, and thalamus are also of critical importance to learning, memory and attention. Abnormalities in their functioning may relate to deficits in forming conditioned fear responses and the failure to learn from experience that characterizes criminal and violent offenders (Raine, 1993). The amygdala additionally plays a role in the recognition of affective and socially-significant stimuli, with destruction of the amygdala in animals resulting in a lack of fear and in man in a reduction in autonomic arousal (Raine et al., 1997). Thus, abnormalities in the amygdala could be relevant to a fearlessness theory of violence based on psychophysiological findings of reduced autonomic arousal in offenders (Raine et al., 1990).

4. POTENTIAL ARTIFACTS AND ETIOLOGY

Could all of these findings possibly be artifacts, with some difference between the groups other than violence producing the findings? We think not. Six of the murderers were schizophrenic, but we controlled for this by including in the control group six non-violent schizophrenics. Furthermore, groups differences in brain functioning were not found to be a function of group differences in age, sex, handedness, history of head injury, medications, or illegal drug use prior to scanning.

Could it be that murderers had poorer prefrontal functioning because they could not do the task? We checked this by looking at how well the murderers did on the continuous performance task. Interestingly their performance was almost identical to controls, and thus this alternative explanation was ruled out. Yet this parity in performance of the challenge task raises another question. How could the murderers do just as well on the task as controls if they have a dysfunction to a part of the brain that is critical to performing the task? We think that the answer may lie in the fact that one brain area, the occipital cortex (visual areas 17 and 18), was *more* activated in murderers than controls. Perhaps the murderers recruited this visual brain area into action to help them preform the visual task and compensate for the poor prefrontal functioning.

We believe this study is important because it constitutes the first evidence from brain imaging to show that the brains of a large sample of murderers are functionally different to normals. There were multisite deficits in the murderers, and although prefrontal deficits have also characterized other disorders such as schizophrenia and depression, studies of these and other psychiatric disorders have never reported this specific pattern of findings involving the prefrontal cortex, corpus callosum, angular gyrus, amygdala, hippocampus, and thalamus, perhaps suggesting a unique signature to this behavioral condition.

Importantly, causality has not been established. It is possible for example that prefrontal dysfunction does not cause violence, but that instead living a violent way of life (including substance abuse and being involved in fights) causes the brain dysfunction that we observed. On the other hand, no previous study has shown that factors like substance abuse and head injuries produce the specific profile of brain deficits that we observed in this group. While we controlled for schizophrenia, it is possible that other psychiatric disorders in the control group could contribute to the findings, although it should be remembered that this specific pattern of brain deficits has never been reported before in any psychiatric group.

If the brain deficits do directly contribute to violence, what causes them? It is possible that they are caused by environmental factors. Although we controlled for a history of head injury, more subtle acts early in life could contribute to brain dysfunction in the murderers. For example, research has shown that violent offenders are more likely to come from abusive homes. If a baby is roughly shaken repeatedly, there can be laceration of the white fibers that link the prefrontal cortex with other brain structures, effectively cutting off the prefrontal regulatory control from the rest of the brain. Thus, it is possible that early infant abuse may have contributed to prefrontal deficits in the murderers. Drug and alcohol abuse may play a contributory, though not total, role. Conversely, the real culprit may be genetics. Although the definitive studies have not been conducted, it is possible that there is a heritable basis to prefrontal functioning, and behavioral and molecular genetic studies are increasingly implicating genetics as a contributory role to crime and violence.

5. PREDATORY VERSUS AFFECTIVE MURDERERS

Do prefrontal deficits especially characterize impulsive, reactive, emotional murderers? Newspapers frequently make reference to the "cold-blooded" predator who dispassionately despatches his victim with little or no emotion. These individuals are contrasted with the passionate, hot-headed individual who kills in a moment of unbridled emotion. Is the predatory killer more controlled and regulated in terms of brain functioning, and is the affective murderer who kills in a moment of passion lacking such brain regulation and control? Animal research has for a long time shown that there are different neural pathways underlying on the one hand predatory or instrumental aggression, versus on the other hand affective or defensive aggression (Mirsky and Siegel, 1994). Imaging research in humans is now beginning to show that the same may be true in humans, at least with respect to that form of aggression that leads to homicide.

In a recent study, we divided our murderers into either "predatory" or "affective" murderers (Raine et al., 1998). The predatory murderers were regulated and controlled, tended to have planned their murder, were lacking in affect, and were more likely to attack a stranger. Conversely the affective murderers showed much less planning to their acts, which were more likely to take place in a domestic context, and were characterized by a high degree of emotion. Some murderers could not be assigned to either of these categories with complete confidence, but in total we were able to assign 15 of the 41 murderers to the predatory group and 9 to the affective group.

The outcome of the study is shown in Figure 2. It shows that the affective murderer shows a lack of prefrontal functioning which would normally form the regulatory control over aggressive impulses. Conversely, the regulated, controlled predatory killer shows relatively good prefrontal functioning, consistent with the role of an intact prefrontal cortex in allowing him to regulate his behavior for nefarious ends. What this finding does not explain is why the predatory murderer is murderous in the first place. The reason may in part lie in subcortical structures. Both groups of murderers were found to have higher functioning of the right subcortex (defined as the midbrain, amygdala, hippocampus, and thalamus) compared to controls. We speculate that excessive subcortical activity may predispose to an aggressive temperament in both groups, but whereas the predatory group have sufficiently good prefrontal functioning to regulate these aggressive impulses in a way to bully and manipulate others to achieve their desired goals, affectively violent individuals lack this prefrontal modulatory control over their impulses, resulting in more impulsive, dysregulated, aggressive outbursts.

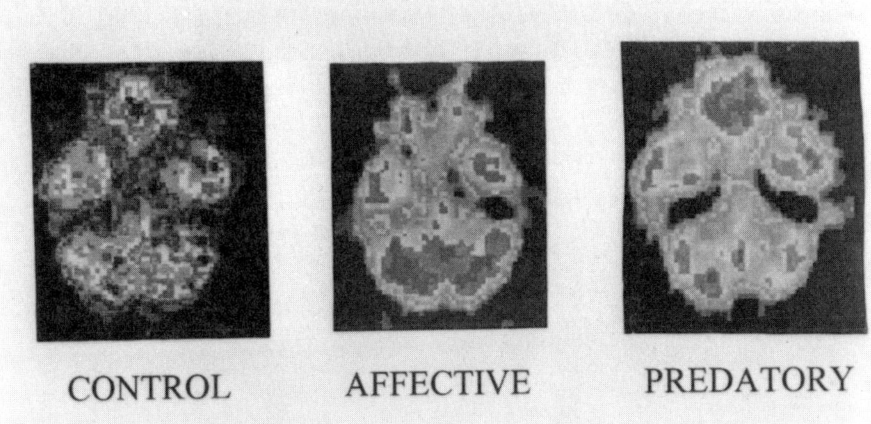

Figure 2. PET scan of normal control (left), affective murderer (middle), and predatory murderer (right) illustrating reduced prefrontal functioning in the affective murderer. Color version of figure appears following page 38.

6. EFFECT OF THE HOME ENVIRONMENT ON BRAIN-VIOLENCE RELATIONSHIPS

How do psychosocial deficits moderate the relationship between prefrontal dysfunction and violence? Perhaps in these cases, the real culprit is not poor family functioning but poor brain functioning.

We recently tested this hypothesis by dividing our sample of murderers up into those who came from relatively good home backgrounds, and those who came from relatively bad home backgrounds (Raine et al., 1998). In this study, ratings of psychosocial deprivation took into account early physical abuse, sexual abuse, neglect, extreme poverty, foster home placement, having a criminal parent, severe family conflict, and a broken home. Twelve murderers were identified as having evidence of significant psychosocial deprivation, whereas 26 were viewed as having minimal evidence of such deprivation.

The results of the study are illustrated in Figure 3 which shows the scan of a normal control (left), a murderer from a bad home (middle), and a murderer from a relatively good home (right). In this case, the odd man out was the murderer from the *good* home. While the deprived murderer shows relatively good prefrontal functioning, it is the non-deprived murderer who shows the characteristic lack of prefrontal functioning. In particular, we found that murderers from good homes had a 14.2% reduction in the functioning of the right orbitofrontal cortex, a brain area that is of particular interest. Damage to this brain area in previously well-controlled adults results in personality and emotional deficits that parallel criminal psychopathic behavior, or what Damasio and colleagues has termed "acquired sociopathy" (Damasio, 1994).

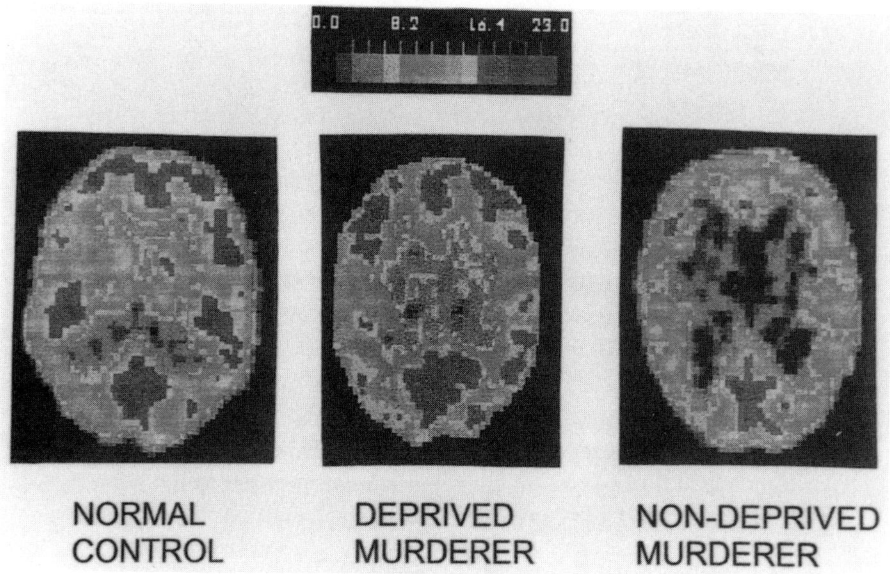

Figure 3. PET scan of normal control (left), murderer from deprived home background (middle) and murderer from benign home background (right) illustrating reduced prefrontal functioning in the non-socially deprived murderer. Color version of figure appears following page 38.

These findings are at one level counter-intuitive, but from another perspective they make some sense. If a seriously violent offender comes from a bad home environment, then it seems likely that the cause of their violence is due to that bad environment. But if they come from a good home background, then environmental causation seems less likely and instead biological deficits may be a better explanation. Consistent with these brain imaging findings, previous research has shown that poor fear conditioning in schoolchildren is related to antisocial behavior especially in those from a *good* home environment (Raine and Venables, 1981). That is, the biological deficit (poor conditioning) is found in those who *lack* a social predisposition to antisocial behavior. Perhaps not surprisingly, it is the right orbitofrontal cortex that has been found to play an important role in the development of fear conditioning.

7. STRUCTURAL PREFRONTAL DEFICITS IN VIOLENT OFFENDERS IN SOCIETY

7.1. Pseudo-psychopathic personality and prefrontal damage

There are three important limitations to our previous functional imaging research. First, the sample is very selected, consisting of murderers pleading not guilty by reason of insanity, an unusual but nevertheless very important subgroup of seriously violent offenders of particular importance in forensic psychiatry. An important question concerns whether prefrontal deficits are also found in offenders who commit less restricted and severe forms of violence such as assault, rape, and robbery. Second, while we found functional deficits to the prefrontal cortex, it is not known whether there are physical, structural deficits which underlie this poor functioning. Third, our sample was institutionalized, and a question is raised as to whether prefrontal deficits could be found in non-institutionalized violent offenders, that is, violent offenders in the community.

We have recently completed a study of structural prefrontal deficits in violent offenders who operate in the community in Los Angeles (Raine et al., 1999). The starting point for this research lies with studies of neurological patients which have provided provocative insights into which brain mechanisms, when damaged, may predispose some individuals towards irresponsible, antisocial, and psychopathic-like behavior. Ranging from single case studies (Damasio et al., 1994) to series of neurological patients (Damasio et al., 1990; Stuss and Benson, 1986), those who have suffered demonstrable damage to both gray and white matter within the prefrontal region of the brain proceed to acquire an antisocial, psychopathic-like personality. These patients also show autonomic arousal and attention deficits to socially-meaningful events (Damasio, 1994, Damasio et al., 1990), a finding consistent with the role played by the prefrontal cortex in modulating emotion, arousal, and attention (Stuss and Benson, 1986; Davidson, 1993; Raine et al., 1991) and with the somatic marker hypothesis that appropriate autonomic functioning is critical to experiencing emotional states that guide prosocial behavior and good decision-making (Damasio, 1994).

While these "developmental sociopaths" (Damasio, 1994) provide intriguing links between ostensible brain damage and onset of antisocial personalty, it could be argued that these findings have little relevance to life-course persistent offenders (Moffitt, 1993) in the community who have consistent antisocial behavior throughout their lives, and yet have not suffered gross brain damage. It has been speculated that developmental sociopaths possess much more subtle prefrontal dysfunction than the blunt macroscopic damage in the acquired sociopath (Damasio, 1994), but there have been no tests of this hypothesis. Specifically, it is not known whether: (1) antisocial individuals in the community have subtle structural deficits to the prefrontal cortex in the absence of discernable lesions (2) these prefrontal deficits are restricted to gray as opposed to white matter (3) prefrontal structural and autonomic functional deficits are specific to antisocial personality disorder as opposed to other forms of psychopathology (4) autonomic deficits are independent of, or conversely linked to, prefrontal deficits (5) prefrontal and autonomic deficits account for variance in antisocials personality over and above that explained by psychosocial deficits.

7.2. Reduced prefrontal gray matter in antisocial personalities

We recently addressed these five questions by conducting structural MRI on volunteers from the community with antisocial personality disorder and making volumetric assessments of prefrontal gray and white matter (Raine et al., 1998). Skin conductance and heart rate activity during a social stressor was also assessed in addition to psychosocial and demographic risk factors for violence. The 1mm spatial resolution of the scanner allowed us to segment gray from white matter within the prefrontal cortex, allowing us to assess whether there was a specific deficit to gray matter (neurons) as opposed to white matter (nerve fibers) in antisocials. An illustration of the ability to discriminate gray from white matter is shown in Figure 4.

Subjects were drawn from temporary employment agencies in Los Angeles and consisted of 21 males with a diagnosis of Antisocial Personality Disorder, 34 male controls who had neither antisocial personality nor drug / alcohol dependence, and 27 male substance dependent controls who had a lifetime diagnosis of drug or alcohol dependence but not Antisocial Personality Disorder.

The Antisocial Personality Disorder group reported having committed a greater number of serious violent crimes than both Controls and Substance Dependents. Specifically, 52.4% of the Antisocials reported having attacked a stranger and caused bruises or bleeding, with rates of 42.9% for rape, 38.1% for firing a gun at someone, and 28.6% for attempted or completed homicide. Antisocials were more likely than both Controls and Substance Abusers to have been arrested by the police. Antisocials also scored 1.4 SDs above the mean of the Substance Dependents on psychopathy who in turn scored 1.0 SDs higher than Controls. Groups were closely comparable on age, social class, ethnicity, intelligence, handedness, history of head injury, weight, and head circumference but as predicted by recent findings on aggressive children (Raine et al., 1998), antisocials were taller than controls.

The important finding to emphasize is that after controlling for this group difference in height, Antisocials had significantly lower prefrontal gray volumes than both Controls and Substance Dependents. In contrast, groups did not differ on white prefrontal volume, indicating specificity of the deficit to gray matter. Furthermore, Antisocials also showed reduced

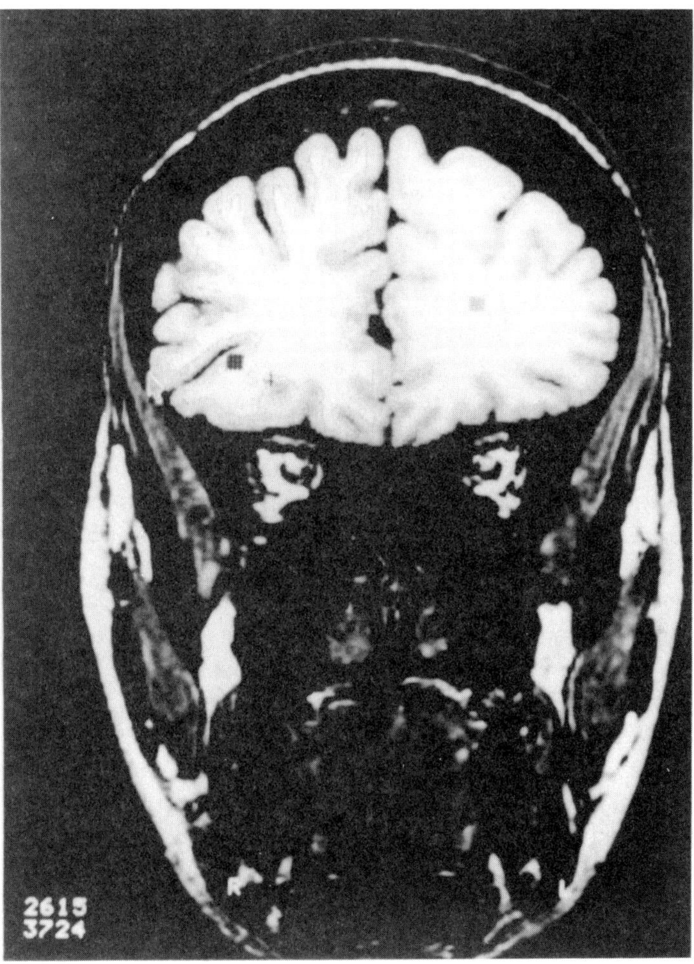

Figure 4. MRI coronal slice of the prefrontal cortex illustrating the seeding program for segmenting gray from white matter. Color version of figure appears following page 38.

autonomic reactivity during the social stressor compared to both Controls and Substance Dependents. When prefrontal gray was expressed as a function of whole brain volume, groups were again found to differ significantly. Further analyses also showed that these brain and autonomic deficits could not be attributed to comorbid affective and schizophrenia-spectrum disorders also present in the Antisocials and which have been shown to have prefrontal structural deficits (Buchsbaum et al., 1997; Raine et al., 1992).

In a logistic regression in which Antisocials were compared to Controls, the three prefrontal and autonomic variables (prefrontal gray / whole brain, heart rate, skin conductance) predicted 50.8% of the variance in group membership, and predicted group membership with an accuracy of 76.9%. Similarly, in predicting Antisocial v.s. Substance Dependence group membership, these measures accounted for 50.2% of the variance, and correctly classified 76.1% of group members.

7.3. Additive effects of biological and psychosocial risk factors

Prefrontal and autonomic deficits were independent of psychosocial deficits in the Antisocial group. This was demonstrated by first entering ten demographic and psychosocial risk factors for antisocial personality (parental social class, early parental divorce, parental verbal arguments, parental criminality, parental physical fights, family size, physical abuse, sexual abuse, raised in an institution, raised by foster parents) into a logistic regression in a single block using forward entry, after which Antisocial versus Control group differences remained significant for prefrontal gray, heart rate, and skin conductance. All comparisons between Antisocial and Substance Dependent groups also remained significant after controlling for psychosocial measures. These analyses importantly indicate that prefrontal and autonomic deficits in antisocials cannot be attributed to psychosocial deficits.

The prefrontal and autonomic deficits added substantially to the prediction of Antisocial vs. Control group membership over and above psychosocial measures. The 10 psychosocial variables in the above logistic regression accounted for 41.3% of the variance. After the additional entry of the three prefrontal gray, heart rate, and skin conductance measures into the regression equation, the amount of group variance explained increased significantly to 76.7%. Prediction of group membership increased from 73.0% correctly classified to 88.5% after including prefrontal and autonomic measures. Similarly, in a comparison of Antisocial versus Substance Dependent groups, the psychosocial variables explained 23.8% of the variance, which increased significantly to 60.0% after entry of the three prefrontal and autonomic variables. Accuracy of group prediction increased from 71.4% to 82.6%.

7.4. Prefrontal structural deficits in psychopathy

To what extent do the above findings on structural prefrontal deficits in antisocial personality disorder apply to psychopathic personality disorder, a related but somewhat different construct? To address this question, subjects were divided into 3 groups on the basis of their scores on the Psychopathy Checklist (PCL; Hare, 1991). The low Psychopathy group was defined as subjects falling into the bottom third of the distribution on PCL scores (range 0-14) while the high psychopathy group fell into the top third of scores (range 23-40).

The High Psychopathy group had significantly lower prefrontal gray / whole brain ratios than the Low Psychopathy group. This reduction existed both for the left hemisphere and the right hemisphere. On the other hand, while the High Psychopathy group had lower skin conductance activity during the stress task than the Low Psychopathy group, the group difference for heart rate was only marginally significant.

7.5. Interpretation of structural prefrontal deficits

The above structural MRI study establishes for the first time the existence of a subtle structural deficit in the prefrontal cortex of antisocial, violent, psychopathic-like individuals who operate in the community. It also extends previous work which has observed pseudo-psychopathic behavior in neurological patients with observable lesions affecting both gray and white matter by showing that a much less observable volume reduction, specific to prefrontal gray, is associated with antisocial personality disorder in this community sample. The Antisocial group had an 11.0% reduction in prefrontal gray compared to Controls, and a 13.9% reduction compared to the Substance Dependent group. Nevertheless, this deficit is virtually imperceptible at a clinical radiological level, with group differences translating to less than half a pixel. Because to our knowledge there has not been a previous MRI study of any antisocial, violent, or psychopathic group, these findings document for the first time the presence of brain deficits in antisocial, psychopathic-like offenders.

What are the mechanisms and processes through which prefrontal and autonomic deficits could predispose to antisocial personality disorder? First, patients with prefrontal damage fail to give anticipatory autonomic responses to choice options that are risky, and make bad choices even when they are aware of the more advantageous response option (Bechara et al., 1997). This inability to reason and decide advantageously in risky situations is likely to contribute to the impulsivity, rule-breaking, and reckless, irresponsible behavior that make up four of the seven traits of antisocial personality disorder. Second, the prefrontal cortex is part of a neural circuit that plays a central role in fear conditioning and stress responsivity (Hugdahl, 1998;

Frysztak & Neafsey, 1991). Poor conditioning is theorized to be associated with poor conscience development (Raine, 1993), and individuals who are less autonomically responsive to aversive stimuli such as social criticism during childhood would be less susceptible to socializing punishments, and hence become predisposed to antisocial behavior. Experiments have repeatedly confirmed that antisocial groups show poor fear conditioning (Raine, 1993). Third, the prefrontal cortex is involved in the regulation of arousal (Dahl, 1998; Hellige, 1993), and deficits in autonomic and central nervous system arousal in antisocials have been viewed as facilitating a stimulation-seeking, antisocial behavioral response to compensate for such underarousal.

8. PHILOSOPHICAL, SPIRITUAL, LEGAL, AND SOCIETAL IMPLICATIONS OF IMAGING RESEARCH

At a scientific level, brain imaging studies on violent, psychopathic offenders are beginning to elucidate the neural networks that may be dysfunctional in these populations. But what are the broader, societal implications that brain imaging studies like these have for society ?

8.1. Philosophical implications

At a philosophical level, imaging work on violence and psychopathy raises the question of whether all of us have freedom of will in the strict sense of the work. If some individuals have damaged brains, can they be said to be fully in control of their actions and cognitions? Do they have complete freedom of will, or does the brain damage place constraints on such freedom? At one extreme, many theologians, philosophers, and scientists would argue that, barring exceptional circumstances such as severe physical and mental illness, each and every one of us has full control over our actions. We choose whether to commit sin or not, and thus our criminal actions (sins) are a product of a will that is under our full control. At the other extreme, some scientists take a more reductionist approach and eschew the idea of a disembodied soul that has its own free will. Francis Crick, for example, believes that free will is nothing more than a large assembly of neurons (probably involving the anterior cingulate cortex), and that under a certain set of assumptions it would be possible to build a machine that would believe it has free will (Crick, 1994).

I would instead argue for a middle ground between these two extremes. I suspect that freedom of will lies on a continuum, with some people having almost complete freedom in their actions, while others have relatively little freedom of will. Rather than viewing intent in black and white, all-or-nothing terms as the law (with a few exceptions) does, it is likely that there are shades of gray, with most of us lying between the extremes. I would argue that early social, biological, and genetic mechanisms play substantial roles in shaping freedom of will (Raine, 1993) and that for some, freedom of will is constrained early in life due to brain dysfunction beyond their control. Brain dysfunction would be a primary process in constraining free will.

8.2. Criminal-justice implications

If brain deficits make it more likely that a person commits violence, and if the cause of the brain deficits was not under the control of the individual, then the question becomes whether or not that person should be held fully responsible for their crimes. In the U.S., many states have the death penalty. Should we execute murderers when we suspect that a pre-existing brain deficit may have made a significant contribution to their actions? Society needs to be protected, and unless the brain deficit can be reversed, such individuals may need to be institutionalized for the rest of their lives. Yet if there is a high probability that brain dysfunction contributed significantly to the act of violence in question, perhaps such even callous, psychopathic offenders should not be executed for their crimes.

It could be countered that despite possessing risk factors for violence which were beyond their control, such offenders need to take responsibility for these predispositions. Although alcoholism is a disease state, society expects that alcoholics should be aware of the fact that they suffer from the disease of alcoholism, take appropriate steps to protect others from the negative effects of their illness, and take responsibility for their actions. Similarly, the person at risk for violence needs to recognize the risk factors that make him dangerous, and take preventive steps to ensure that they do not harm others. They may have risk factors, but they still have responsibility and they still have free will.

The problem with this counter-argument is that responsibility and self-reflection are not disembodied, ethereal processes, but are rooted firmly in the brain. Patients who have damage to the ventromedial prefrontal cortex are known to become irresponsible, lack self-discipline, and fail to reflect on the consequences of their actions (Damasio, 1994). The very mechanism that subserves the ability to take responsibility for ones' actions is damaged in the violent, psychopathic offender. He is no longer able to reflect on his behavior, check his impulses, modify his behavior as a function of changing situational demands, and therefore is unable to take full responsibility for his predispositions.

Should brain scan data be used in courts of law? Brain scan data have frequently been used in the sentencing stage of the trials of capital cases after the defendant had been found guilty and when all possible grounds for mitigation and sentence reduction may be reviewed. But in a landmark case in 1991 brain scan data was for the first time successfully used in the guilt phase of a homicide trial resulting in much-lighter sentence for manslaughter. In this case, a man who strangled his wife and threw her out of the 12th floor of their Manhatten apartment block (D'Agincourt, 1993). A PET scan of the defendant subsequently found poor functioning in the left frontal and temporal brain regions.

8.3. Societal implications

There are multiple political, theological, and moral issues that give rise to objections to the application of biological findings on violence to the legal system (Raine, 1993). At a political level, biological research on violence is often unpopular with both the right and the left sides of the political spectrum. The conservative right is worried that biological research will be used to let vicious offenders off the hook, encouraging a soft approach to crime control. On the other hand, the liberal left is concerned that brain scan technology will ultimately be used to scan the brains of innocent individuals and lock up those with the profile of a violent offender before they have a chance to commit crime. Theologians don't like the idea that biology puts constraints on the individual's freedom of will because their egalitarian belief is that God has made all us equally able to embrace his son Jesus and reject sin. At a broad, moral level, most of us feel that offenders just have to be punished if they do wrong - it would be morally wrong not to. And practically, what would happen in a society where serious crimes were excused because of bad brains? Surely this would become license to kill without conscience and consequence?

Brain imaging research on violence and psychopathy is troubling to some because it challenges the way we conceptualize crime. It questions our treatment of violent psychopaths in just the same way that we now look back 200 years and question the way in which the mentally ill were kept in shackles and chains, treated little better than animals. The history of civilization has shown that as time progresses, society becomes more ennobled, wiser, and humane. In 200 years from now, will we have reconceptualized recidivistic repeat serious criminal behavior as a clinical disorder with its roots in early social, biological, and genetic forces beyond the individual's control? Will we look back aghast at our current practices of execution and inhumane treatment of seriously violent offenders? Will we view this execution of prisoners as barbaric and unjustified as we now view the burning of witches?

I would like to think that we will, but perhaps the one thing that will not change in society is our gut reaction to crime. There are many reasons why we have been successful as a species, but one is that we have created effective mechanisms to shut out those in our midst with antisocial, violent, and psychopathic tendencies. For that reason, nothing may change with respect to how we conceptualize and deal with criminal violence. Yet I believe this would be an enormous mistake. Brain imaging, together with other biological research, is beginning to give us new and at times dramatic insights into what makes up the violent, psychopathic-like offender. Hopefully these early findings might lead us to rethink our approach to violence and psychopathy and goad us into obtaining new answers to the causes and cures of crime while we continue to protect society and the victims of violence.

REFERENCES

Bechara, A.; Damasio, H.; Tranel, D. & Damasio, A. R. (1997): "Deciding advantageously before knowing the advantageous strategy", *Science*, 275, pp. 1293-1294.

Benson, D. F. & Miller, B. L. (1997): "Frontal lobe mechanisms of aggression", in J. S. Grisolía, J. Sanmartín, J. L. Luján & S. Grisolía (eds.), *Violence: From biology to society*, Amsterdam, Elsevier, pp. 35-42.

Buchsbaum, M. S. et al. (1997): "Ventricular volume and asymmetry in schizotypal personality disorder and schizophrenia assessed with magnetic resonance imaging", *Schizophrenia Research*, 27, pp. 45-53.

Crick, F. (1994): *The astonishing hypothesis: The scientific search for the soul,* New York, Touchstone.

D'Agincourt, L. (1993): "PET findings support insanity defense case", *Diagnostic imaging*, 15, pp. 45-50.

Dahl, R. E. (1998): "Development and psychopathology", in E. A. Farber & M. Hertzig (eds), *Annual progress in child psychiatry and child development*, Bristol PA, Brunner/Mazel, pp. 3-28.

Damasio, A. R. (1994): *Descartes' Error: Emotion, reason, and the human brain,* New York, Grosset/Putnam.

Damasio, H.; Grabowski, T.; Frank, R.; Galaburda, A. M. & Damasio, A. R. (1994): "The return of Phineas Gage: Clues about the brain from a skull of a famous patient", *Science*, 264, pp. 1102-1105.

Damasio, A. R.; Tranel, D. & Damasio, H. (1990): "Individuals with psychopathic behavior caused by frontal damage fail to respond autonomically to social stimuli", *Behavioral and Brain Research*, 41, pp. 81-94.

Davidson, R. J. (1993): "Parsing affective space: Perspectives from neuropsychology and psychophysiology", Neuropsychology, 7, pp. 464-475.

Davidson, R. J. & Fox, N. A. (1989): "Frontal brain asymetry predicts infants' response to maternal separation", *Journal of Abnormal Psychology*, 98, pp. 127-131.

Denenberg, V. H.; Gall, J. S.; Berrebi, A. & Yutzey, D. A. (1986): "Callosal mediation of cortical inhibition in the lateralized rat brain", *Brain Research*, 397, pp. 327-332.

Dodge, K. A.; Price, J. M. & Bachorowski, J. A. (1990): "Hostile attributional biases in severely aggressive adolescents", *Journal of Abnormal Psychology*, 99, pp. 385-392.

Frysztak, R. J. & Neafsey, E. J. (1991): "The effect of medial frontal cortex lesions on respiration, 'freezing', and ultrasonic vocalizations during conditioned emotional responses in rats", *Cerebral Cortex*, 1, pp. 418-425.

Fuster, J. M. (1989): *The prefrontal cortex: Anatomy, physiology, and neuropsychology of the frontal lobe,* (2nd ed.), New York, Raven Press.

Garbanati, J. A.; Sherman, G. F.; Rosen, G. D.; Hofmann, M. J.; Yutzey, D. A. & Denenberg, V. H. (1993): "Handling in infancy, brain laterality and muricide in rats", *Behavioral and Brain Research*, 7, pp. 351-359.

Grisolia, J.S. (1997): "Temporal lobe mechanisms and violence", in J. S. Grisolía, J. Sanmartín, J. L. Lujan & S. Grisolia (eds), *Violence: From biology to society*, Amsterdam, Elsevier, pp. 43-52.

Gur, R. C.; Ragland, J. D.; Resnick, S. M.; Skolnick, B. E.; Jaggi, J.; Muencz, L. & Gur, R. E. (1994): "Lateralized increases in cerebral blood flow during performance of verbal and spatial tasks: relationship with performance level", *Brain and Cognition*, 24, pp. 244-258.

Goyer, P. F.; Andreason, P. J.; Semple, W. E.; Clayton, A. H.; King, A. C.; Compton-Toth, B. A.; Schulz, S. C. & Cohen, R.M. (1994): "Positron-emission tomography and personality disorders", *Neuropsychopharmacology*, 10, pp. 21-28.

Hare, R. D. (1991): *The Hare Psychopathy Checklist – Revised*, New York, Multi-Health Systems.

Hellige, J. (1993): *Hemisphere asymmetry: What's right and what's left*, Cambridge, Harvard University Press.

Henry, B. & Moffitt, T. E. (1997): "Neuropsychological and neuroimaging studies of juvenile delinquency and adult criminal behavior", in J. Breiling, D. M. Stoff & J. D. Maser, *Handbook of antisocial behavior*, New York, Wiley, pp. 280-288.

Hugdahl, K. (1998): "Cortical control of human classical conditioning: Autonomic and positron emission tomography data", *Psychophysiology*, 35, pp. 170-178.

Intrator, J.; Hare, R.; Stritzke, P.; Brichtswein, K.; Dorfman, D.; Harpur, T. Bernstein, D.; Handelsman, L.; Schaefer, C.; Keilp, J.; Rosen, J. & Machac, J. (1997): "A brain imaging (single photon emission computerized tomography) study of semantic and affective processing in psychopaths", *Biological Psychiatry*, 42, pp. 96-103.

Kuruoglu, A. C.; Arikan, Z.; Karatas, M.; Arac, M. & Isik, E. (1996): "Single photon emission computerized tomography in chronic alcoholism: Antisocial Personality Disorder may be associated with decreased frontal perfusion", *British Journal of Psychiatry*, 169, pp. 348-354.

Mirsky, A. F. & Siegel, A. (1994): "The neurobiology of violence and aggression", in A. J. Reiss, K. A. Miczek & J. A. Roth (eds.), *Understanding and preventing violence. Vol. 2. Biobehavioral influences*, Washington D.C., National Academy Press, pp. 59-172.

Moffitt, T. E. (1993): "Adolescence-limited and life-course persistent antisocial behavior: A developmental taxonomy", *Psychological Review*, 100, pp. 674-701.

Raine, A. (1993): *The Psychopathology of crime: Crime behavior as a clinical disorder*, San Diego, Academic Press.

Raine, A. & Buchsbaum, M. S. (1996): "Violence and brain imaging", in D. M. Stoff & R. B. Cairns (eds.), *Neurobiological approaches to clinical aggression research*, Mahwah NJ, Lawrence Erlbaum, pp. 195-218.

Raine, A.; Buchsbaum, M. S.; Stanley, J.; Lottenberg, S.; Abel, L. & Stoddard, J. (1994): "Selective reductions in pre-frontal glucose metabolism in murderers", *Biological Psychiatry*, 36, 365-373. (También reeditado in Talbott, J. A. (1996) (ed.): *The Yearbook of Psychiatry and Applied Mental Health*, St. Louis, Mosby) (see also correspondence in (1995): *Biological Psychiatry*, 38, pp. 342-343).

Raine, A.; Buchsbaum, M. S. & La Casse, L. (1997): "Brain abnormalities in murderers indicated by positron emission tomography", *Biological Psychiatry*, 42, pp. 495-508.

Raine, A.; Reynolds, C.; Venables, P. H.; Mednick, S. A. & Farrington, D. P. (1998): "Fearlessness, stimulation-seeking, and large body size at age 3 years as early predispositions to childhood aggression at age 11 years", *Archives of General Psychiatry*, 55, pp. 745-751.

Raine, A.; Reynolds, G. & Sheard, C. (1991): "Neuroanatomical mediators of electrodermal activity in normal human subjects: A magnetic resonance imaging study", *Psychophysiology*, 28, pp. 548-555.

Raine, A.; Sheard, S.; Reynolds, G. P. & Lencz, T. (1992): "Pre-frontal structural and functional deficits associated with individual differences in schizotypal personality", *Schizophrenia Research*, 7, pp. 237-247.

Raine, A.; Stoddard, J.; Bihrle, S. & Buchsbaum, M. S. (1998): "Prefrontal glucose deficits in murderers lacking psychosocial deprivation", *Neuropsychiatry, Neuropsychology, and Behavioral Neurology*, 11, pp. 1-7.

Raine, A.; Meloy, J. R.; Bihrle, S.; Stoddard, J.; Lacasse, L. & Buchsbaum, M. S. (1998): "Reduced prefrontal and increased subcortical brain functioning assessed using positron emission tomography in predatory and affective murderers", *Behavioral Sciences and the Law*, 16, pp. 319-332.

Raine, A. & Venables, P. H. (1981): "Classical conditioning and socialization - A biosocial interaction?", *Personality and Individual Differences*, 2, pp. 273-283.

Raine, A.; Venables, P. H. & Williams, M. (1990): "Relationships between CNS and ANS measures of arousal at age 15 and criminality at age 24", *Archives of General Psychiatry*, 47, pp. 1003-1007.

Seidenwurm, D.; Pounds, T. R.; Globus, A. & Valk, P. E. (1997): "Temporal lobe metabolism in violent subjects: Correlation of imaging and neuropsychiatric findings", *American Journal of Neuroradiology*, 18, pp. 625-631.

Stuss, D. T. & Benson, D. F. (1986): *The frontal lobes*, New York, Raven Press.

Volkow, N. D.; Tancredi, L. R.; Grant, C.; Gillespie, H.; Valentine, A.; Mullani, N.; Wang, G. J. & Hollister, L. (1995): "Brain glucose metabolism in violent psychiatric patients: A preliminary study", *Psychiatry Research – Neuroimaging*, 61, pp. 243-253.

Chapter 3

EMOTIONAL PROCESSES IN PSYCHOPATHY

Christopher J. Patrick
Department of Psychology, University of Minnesota, USA

1. EMOTIONAL PROCESSES IN PSYCHOPATHY

Emotion is important to understanding aggression and violence because it is the force that drives behavior. Individuals who behave violently usually do so because they are moved to do so by strong emotions. However, empirical research indicates that psychopaths are highly aggressive, but also detached and unemotional. To resolve this apparent contradiction, it is necessary to consider that there may be different forms of aggression and different aspects of psychopathy. This paper outlines a theoretical model of emotion, and a methodology (the startle-probe technique), for investigating basic emotional processes in normal and abnormal individuals. Recent research of this kind in criminal offender populations suggests that the detached, predatory style of the "true" psychopath is related to a weakness in the defensive system of the brain that governs negative emotional response. In turn, this emotional weakness is related to a particular set of temperament traits, and specific forms of aggressive behavior.

2. THEORY OF EMOTION

During the mid-1900's, psychological theories of emotion and techniques for measuring emotion assumed that a single arousal system existed in the brain (Lindsley, 1951). The basic idea was that sympathetic nervous system activity and emotional arousal increased as brain arousal increased, and that autonomic (skin conductance, heart rate) and cortical (EEG) activity could be used to measure overall activation. However, a weakness of this single arousal system model was that it did not account for obvious differences among emotional states.

To deal with this problem, Donald Hebb (1955) developed a two-factor theory in which emotional states were described as varying in direction as well as intensity of activation. Hebb believed that the direction of emotional expression was determined by stimuli in the environment that called for one

Violence and Psychopathy, edited by Raine & Sanmartin,
Kluwer Academic/Plenum Publishers, New York, 2001.

type of action or another. For example, an animal could respond to a threatening intruder by running away if that option was available, or by attacking if it was not. In a similar manner, social psychologist Stanley Schachter (1964) theorized that differences in the experience and expression of emotion are determined by the cognitive interpretation or label that is attached to a general state of arousal, due to the features of the situation in which the arousal is elicited.

The research described in this paper draws on the ideas of these early emotion theorists together with more recent developments in emotion research and brain science. This work emphasizes the idea that emotion involves more than one activation system, and processing at different levels of the brain (Lang, 1995; Patrick, in press; Stritzke, Lang, & Patrick, 1996). In contrast to the single-arousal model, it is assumed that different emotional states serve different behavioral functions. Through the process of natural selection, separate brain systems evolved to control different categories of survival-related behaviors—those related to avoiding danger, and those related to gaining reward. Stimuli in the environment that signal reward or punishment activate one or the other brain system, producing a state of readiness to either approach or avoid. These states of readiness can be viewed as the essence of emotion (Izard, 1993; Lang, 1995; Plutchik, 1984). In this sense, "motivation" involves preparation for adaptive action.

Several types of evidence support the idea that emotions involve activation in one of two basic brain systems, an aversive (negative emotion) system controlling defensive reactions, and an appetitive (positive) system controlling approach behaviors (Gray, 1987; Lang, 1995). Schneirla (1959) concluded from his studies of various animal species that approach and avoidance are the most basic forms of behavioral expression. Similarly, Konorski (1967) identified two main categories of external reflexes in mammals, appetitive and defensive. McLean (1958), building on earlier work by Papez (1937), proposed that the basic emotion centers in the brain are subcortical structures that developed early in evolution to control survival behaviors related to approach and avoidance. Another finding that is consistent with this idea of two motivational systems is that statistical analyses of mood or emotion words have consistently revealed two major factors or dimensions (Tellegen, 1985; Russell & Mehrabian, 1977).

However, it is important to recognize that these basic approach and avoidance systems communicate with other areas of the brain, including systems that control attention, memory, and thought (LeDoux, 1995). Because of this, emotional reactions can be influenced by prior learning, by ongoing information processing, and by the overall characteristics of a situation. For example, a negative emotional reaction can be elicited by a simple sensory cue (e.g.,. a light that signals shock) or by a complex symbolic stimulus (e.g., a language description of a frightening event), and the reaction can lead to different behavioral expressions (e.g., freezing, flight, attack) depending upon the overall situation.

To summarize, emotion involves processing at both lower subcortical and higher cortical levels (Stritzke et al., 1996). This model of emotional processing is consistent with earlier theories that emphasized the impact of cognitive factors on emotional state (e.g., Schachter, 1964; Lazarus, 1982). However, the current model assumes that cognitive processes influence the expression of approach or avoidance tendencies, rather than general arousal. Specific emotional states like fear, disgust, and anger (Ekman, 1992; Izard, 1993) can be viewed as defensive reactions that are shaped in characteristic ways by past and present experience (Lang, Bradley, & Cuthbert, 1990). Also, the current model does not assume that cognitive processing has to occur before emotion is elicited, or vice versa (Lazarus, 1984; Zajonc, 1984). Instead, the model allows for the possibility of either sequence (Lang, 1994; LeDoux, 1995; Öhman, 1993; Zajonc, 1980).

3. EMOTION, ATTENTION, AND STARTLE REFLEX MODULATION

A well-established finding in normal humans is that the eye-blink startle reaction to a sudden noise is reliably larger (potentiated) during viewing of emotionally unpleasant pictures (e.g., snakes, dead bodies, aimed guns) in comparison to neutral pictures (e.g., kitchen utensils, neutral faces). On the other hand, the startle reflex is reliably smaller (inhibited) during viewing of pleasant pictures (e.g., happy babies, nude couples) in comparison to neutral (Lang, 1995; see Figure 1).

One way to think about these changes in the protective blink reflex is that they reflect activation of one motivation system or the other by the picture stimulus. Unpleasant pictures activate the defensive system, and the resulting action state matches with the defensive reaction to the aversive noise probe, leading to reflex potentiation. Like a coiled spring, the fear-activated organism is prepared for immediate action—and the effect of the unexpected noise probe is to trigger this action. On the other hand, pleasant pictures elicit a state of attentive approach that opposes the defensive blink reaction to the noise, resulting in a smaller startle response. In this respect, changes in the magnitude of the startle reflex response can be used to infer whether the reaction to an emotional stimulus is positive (appetitive) or negative (defensive).

It has been clearly demonstrated that startle reflex potentiation reflects activation of the defensive system. In both animals and humans, startle potentiation is reliably observed during exposure to threatening stimuli, and the effect is blocked by drugs that reduce anxiety (Davis, 1979; Patrick, Berthot, & Moore, 1996). Furthermore, Davis (1989) showed that fear-

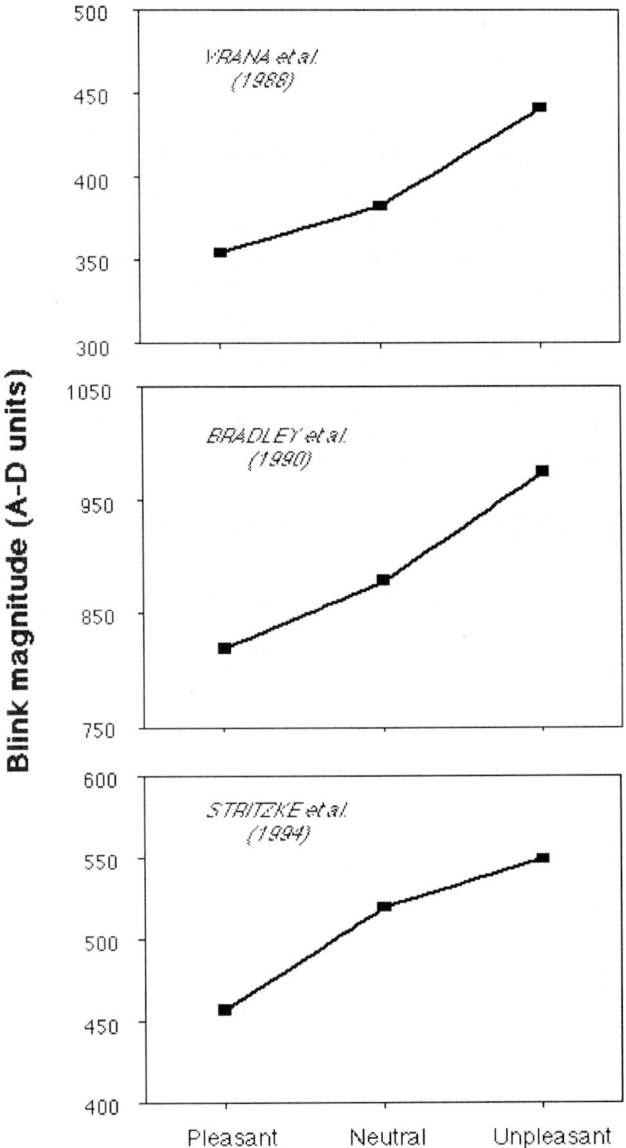

Figure 1. *Mean startle blink magnitude (A-D units) during pleasant, neutral, and unpleasant pictures in three representative studies of normal men and women: Vrana, Spence, and Lang (1988); Bradley, Cuthbert, and Lang (1990); and Stritzke, Patrick, and Lang (1995).*

potentiated startle in animals is mediated by the amygdala (Figure 2), a subcortical structure that is considered to be the core of the defensive motivational system (Fanselow, 1994; LeDoux, 1995).

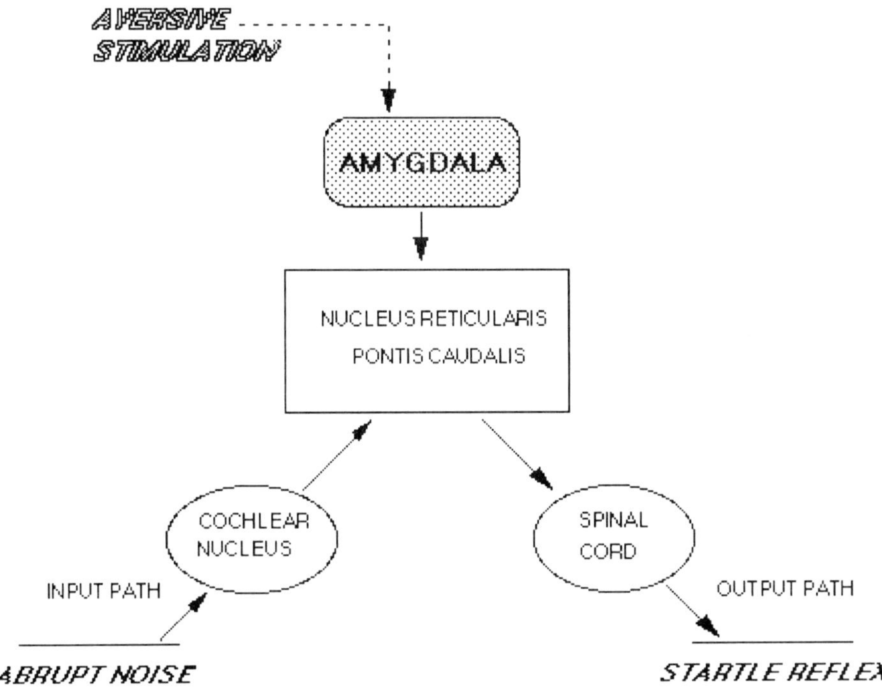

Figure 2. Schematic diagram of the neural circuit that is believed to underlie the startle reflex and its potentiation by fear. The mechanism for fear-potentiated startle is a pathway from the central nucleus of the amygdala to the nucleus reticularis pontis caudalis. This model is based on animal research by Michael Davis and colleagues (cf. Davis, 1986; Davis, 1997).

On the other hand, recent evidence indicates that the inhibition of the blink startle response that occurs during pleasant picture viewing results from greater attention to the picture stimulus. Cuthbert, Bradley, and Lang (1996) measured skin conductance (SC) and blink startle reactions during viewing of pleasant and unpleasant pictures that varied in rated arousal. For both picture types, SC response (a nonspecific measure of activation; Greenwald, Cook, & Lang, 1989) increased in direct relation to picture intensity—that is, as pictures (whether pleasant or unpleasant) became more intense, SC response became larger. For pleasant pictures, startle magnitude decreased continuously with increasing stimulus arousal (i.e., more intense pictures produced greater blink inhibition). However, for unpleasant pictures, the direction of startle magnitude change reversed as pictures became more intense: For pictures of low to moderate intensity, the startle response was inhibited, but higher intensity pictures produced increasing startle potentiation (Figure 3). The explanation was that less intense aversive pictures distracted attention away from the noise probe (Anthony & Graham, 1985), but more intense pictures activated the defensive system, causing startle potentiation.

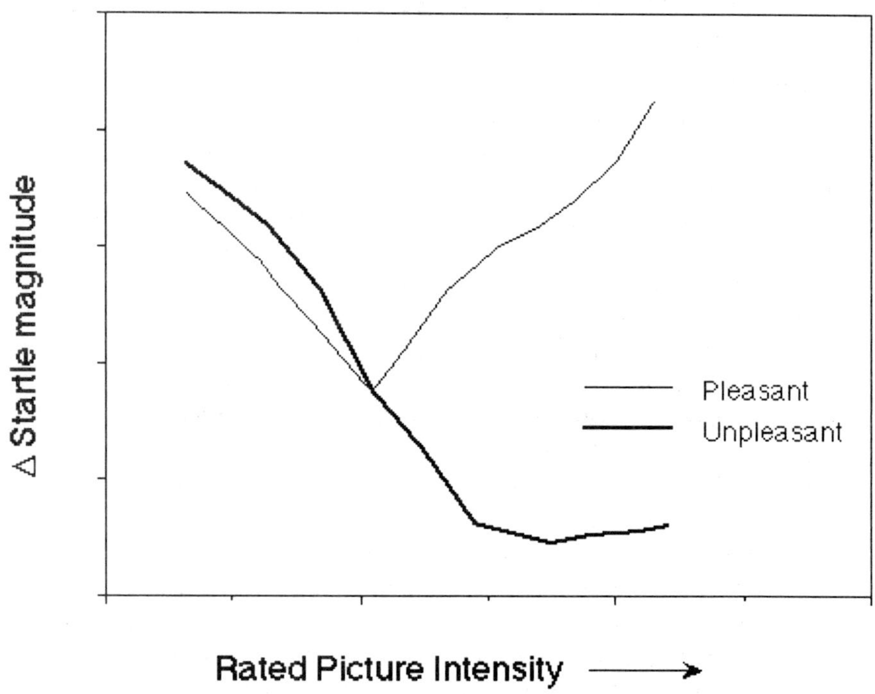

Figure 3. Changes in the magnitude of the blink startle reflex during viewing of pleasant and unpleasant pictures of increasing intensity (adapted from Cuthbert, Bradley, & Lang, 1996).

Based on these and other findings, Lang, Bradley, and Cuthbert (1997) theorized that environmental stimuli with emotional meaning (i.e., that are pleasant or unpleasant) attract greater attention than stimuli that are neutral. However, if the stimuli are aversive, this attentional (orienting) response is replaced by a withdrawal (defensive) response as the stimuli become more intense. This shift from an orienting to a defensive state occurs automatically and in stages. If unpleasant stimuli are moderately intense, orienting and defensive tendencies can both be present at the same time; however, when danger becomes immediate the defensive system takes over completely, resulting in avoidance or attack behavior (Fanselow, 1994; Lang et al.,

1997). This shift from orienting to defense can be viewed as a tradeoff between two basic survival tendencies, reward-related approach and threat-related avoidance. The position of the present paper is that psychopathic individuals have a higher threshold for shifting from orienting to defense than normal individuals. That is, in psychopaths, unpleasant stimuli have to be highly intense for defensive activation to occur.

4. PSYCHOPATHIC PERSONALITY: DIAGNOSTIC FEATURES

The disorder of psychopathy is different from antisocial behavior or criminal deviance. Psychopaths have a specific emotional and interpersonal style that is characterized by an absence of close personal relationships and selfish manipulation of other people. Stated more simply, psychopaths seem to lack the ability to love or to feel guilt. As a consequence of this, the psychopath operates as a social strategist or predator, taking care of his immediate selfish needs without regard for the consequences. The term "primary" (or "true") psychopath has been used to refer to individuals of this type.

Hervey Cleckley (1976) described psychopathy as a "mask of sanity" in which severe emotional deficits are hidden behind an appearance of normal thought and speech. The psychopath looks normal at first, but upon closer examination he is found to be severely lacking in the ability to connect or to empathize with other people. In this regard, Cleckley's diagnostic criteria for psychopathy included the following: low in anxiety; lacks remorse or shame; self-centered and unable to love; lacks major affective reactions, and shows reckless, irresponsible behavior. Cleckley viewed the underlying emotional deviation in psychopathy as something that was present from birth, and which could exist in differing degrees in different people. Thus, his case histories included examples of successful professionals and scholars as well as criminal offenders.

Hare (1980) developed the Psychopathy Checklist (PCL) as a method for identifying Cleckley psychopaths in prison settings. The revised version of the Psychopathy Checklist (PCL-R; Hare, 1991) includes 20 items, each rated on a 0-2 scale (0 = no, 1 = maybe, 2 = yes) on the basis of information collected from a diagnostic interview and from prison files. Scores on the 20 individual items are added together, and total scores of 30 or result in a diagnosis of psychopathy.

Factor analyses of the PCL (Harpur, Hakstian, & Hare, 1988; Harpur, Hare, & Hakstian, 1989) have revealed two major factors or dimensions, which were labeled <u>emotional detachment</u> and <u>antisocial behavior</u> by Patrick, Bradley, & Lang (1993). Factor 1 is marked by items that reflect the core emotional and interpersonal symptoms of psychopathy that Cleckley emphasized. Factor 2 is marked by items describing long term antisocial behavior, including child behavior problems, impulsiveness, irresponsibility, and a lack of long-term goals. The PCL includes one item that deals specifically with anger and aggressiveness ("poor behavioral controls"), and this item loads on the antisocial behavior factor.

The two PCL factors show contrasting relationships with other measures of personality and behavior. Scores on the emotional detachment factor are negatively correlated with self-report anxiety scales and positively related to measures of social dominance, narcissistic personality, and Machiavellianism (Harpur et al., 1989; Hare, 1991). Ratings on the antisocial behavior factor are positively correlated with impulsiveness, sensation seeking, and frequency of criminal offending (Harpur et al, 1989; Hare, 1991), and also alcohol and drug abuse (Smith & Newman, 1990).

Antisocial personality disorder (APD) as described in the fourth edition of the Diagnostic and Statistical Manual of Mental Disorders (DSM-IV; American Psychiatric Association, 1994) is closely related to the behavioral but not the emotional factor of the PCL. This is because the criteria for APD consist mostly of behavioral signs and symptoms (e.g., rule-breaking, recklessness, and aggression in childhood and in adulthood). In prison settings, the base rate of APD (70-80%) is much higher than that of psychopathy as defined by the PCL-R (25-30%). Individuals who show persistent antisocial behavior but who lack the core emotional symptoms of psychopathy are sometimes referred to as "secondary psychopaths." A variety of risk factors, including birth complications, low intelligence, poverty, bad parenting, physical or sexual abuse, and negative peer influence, seem to play a role in this type of antisocial deviance (Lykken, 1995; Raine, 1993).

5. PSYCHOPATHIC PERSONALITY: THEORY AND RESEARCH

Clinical descriptions have emphasized the idea that psychopaths are deviant in emotional reactivity (Cleckley, 1976; Hare, 1991), and a major focus of research in this area has been on how psychopaths differ in their processing of emotional stimuli. Lykken (1957) reported the first empirical evidence that psychopaths defined by Cleckley's criteria were deficient in their ability to develop anxiety responses. Since this paper was published, a good deal of research has focused on the reactivity of psychopaths to situations involving punishment or threat. The most consistent findings have been that psychopaths show (a) lower skin conductance reactivity during anticipation of an aversive event, and (b) poor passive avoidance learning, i.e., a failure to learn to inhibit punished responses (Hare, 1978; Arnett, 1997). More recent studies using the fear-potentiated startle paradigm, reviewed below, have provided direct evidence for a weakness in defensive emotional reactivity among psychopathic offenders.

Other empirical studies have focused on the possibility that psychopathy involves disturbances in attention, or cognitive processing . One hypothesis is that psychopaths are generally less able to process peripheral events when attending to stimuli of immediate interest (Jutai & Hare, 1983; Kosson & Newman, 1986). However, the evidence for this simple "overfocusing" hypothesis is weak (Kosson & Harpur, 1997; Newman & Wallace, 1993). A related idea is that psychopaths fail to process secondary features of a stimulus when their attention is directed toward specified features of that same stimulus; Kosson (1996, 1998) has presented evidence in support of this position. Relatedly, Newman, Schmitt, and Voss (1997) reported that psychopaths showed less interference in a stimulus processing task in which words and pictures of different meanings were presented at the same time.

Other research suggests that psychopathy could involve deviations in both emotion and attention. Christianson, Forth, Hare, Strachan, Lidberg, and Thorell (1996) reported that nonpsychopaths showed poorer memory for a peripheral detail of an accident picture than for a central detail, whereas psychopaths did not show this difference. The authors' interpretation was that psychopaths attended less to the central accident detail because it did not have the same emotional impact on them. Williamson, Harpur, and Hare (1991) reported that psychopaths discriminated pleasant, neutral, and unpleasant words from nonwords as quickly and accurately as nonpsychopaths, but they did not show a difference between neutral and emotional words in either reaction time or early brain potentials (P240, P600). This result indicates that the automatic discrimination between emotional and neutral stimuli that occurs in normal individuals (Lang et al., 1997) is impaired in psychopaths.

6. EMOTION AND STARTLE REFLEX RESPONDING IN CRIMINAL PSYCHOPATHS

Patrick et al. (1993) reported a deviant pattern of startle reactivity in psychopathic prisoners during viewing of pleasant, neutral, and unpleasant pictures. Diagnoses were based on overall scores on Hare's (1991) PCL-R. Noise probes occurred between 3.5 and 5.5 s after picture onset. High PCL-R scorers, in contrast to individuals with low or moderate psychopathy scores, did not show startle potentiation while viewing unpleasant pictures. Instead, the psychopath group showed blink <u>inhibition</u> for both pleasant and unpleasant pictures in comparison to neutral. In light of the animal and human data linking startle potentiation to fear, this pattern suggests that aversive stimuli do not as readily elicit a defensive reaction in psychopaths.

In turn, this finding is consistent with the hypothesis that psychopathy involves a deficit in anxiety or fear (Fowles, 1980; Hare, 1970; Lykken, 1957).

In a subsequent study, Levenston, Patrick, Bradley, and Lang (in press) measured startle responses in male prisoners during viewing of neutral pictures and different categories of aversive and pleasant pictures. The aversive picture categories included direct threat scenes (aimed weapons; threatening attackers) and victim scenes (assaults on others; injured people). The pleasant pictures included erotic scenes (nudes, intimate couples) and risky adventure scenes (e.g., roller coaster, ski jump). Startle noises occurred at varying times during the picture viewing interval.

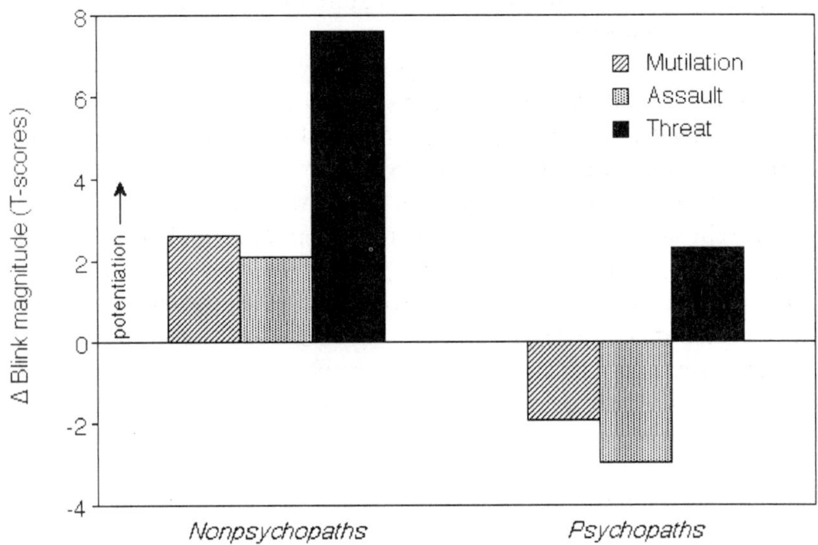

Figure 4. Increase in blink response to startling noises presented during victim (mutilation, assault) and threat pictures, compared to neutral pictures. Results are for two prisoner groups, psychopathic men and nonpsychopathic men. Units are standard T-scores (for details, see Patrick, Bradley & Lang, 1993).

Replicating the findings of Patrick et al. (1993), different startle patterns were observed for high versus low PCL-R scorers: Nonpsychopathic prisoners showed startle potentiation for unpleasant scenes beginning at 800 ms after picture onset, but psychopaths showed blink reflex inhibition for both pleasant and unpleasant pictures compared to neutral. For specific picture categories, nonpsychopaths showed moderate blink potentiation for victim scenes, strong potentiation for threat scenes, and blink inhibition only for erotic pictures (with modest potentiation for adventure scenes). For psychopaths, the blink startle response was inhibited during victim scenes and only weakly potentiated during threat scenes. Psychopaths also showed reliable blink inhibition for both erotic and adventure scenes. (See Figure 4.)

The finding of startle reflex inhibition during victim scenes indicates that psychopaths reacted to these aversive scenes mainly by attending (orienting) to them. In contrast, nonpsychopaths showed moderate startle potentiation during victim pictures, indicating some degree of defensive activation. For the threat pictures, psychopaths showed only weak startle potentiation, whereas nonpsychopaths showed very strong potentiation. These results indicate that an aversive stimulus must be more intense to produce a shift from orienting to defense in psychopaths (Figure 5).

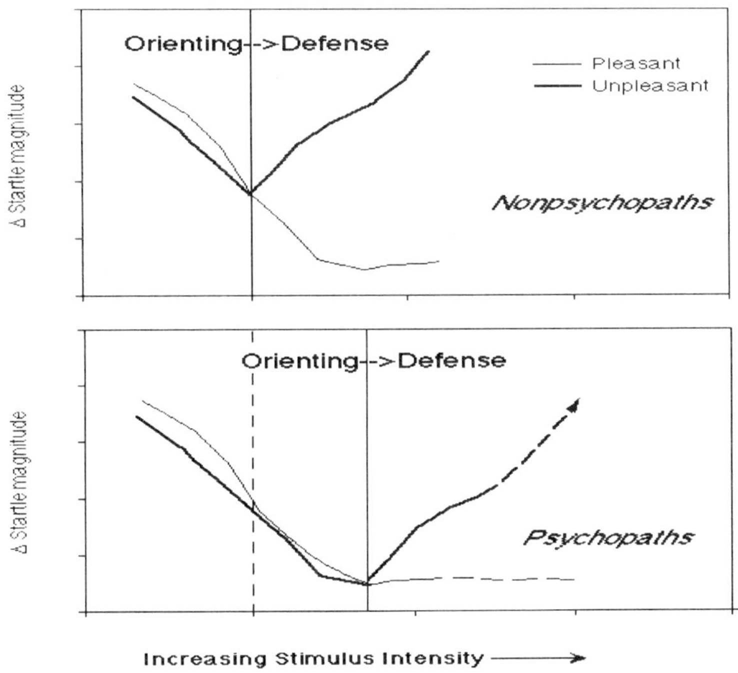

Figure 5. Hypothesized mechanism for reduced startle potentiation during aversive pictures in psychopathic individuals. According to the model, psychopaths have a higher threshold for shifting from attentional orienting to defense (Levenston, Patrick, Bradley, & Lang, in press).

Nonpsychopathic prisoners (like normal men; Levenston & Patrick, 1995) showed evidence of startle potentiation for the less intense victim scenes, but psychopaths showed evidence of potentiation only for the more intense threat scenes.

The group differences for pleasant pictures can be explained in a similar way. Both groups showed blink inhibition for the erotic pictures, which were purely pleasurable. However, the adventure scenes included elements of danger as well as excitement. For these pictures, the nonpsychopaths showed some defensive reactivity (i.e., blink potentiation), whereas psychopaths showed only an attentional reaction (i.e., blink inhibition). Again, this suggests that psychopaths have a higher threshold for shifting from orienting to defense—that is, aversive cues must be more intense to activate a defensive state in these individuals.

7. THE RELATIONSHIP BETWEEN EMOTIONAL DEFICITS AND DIAGNOSTIC FEATURES OF PSYCHOPATHY

In the Patrick et al. (1993) study, abnormal startle reactivity was most evident among individuals who scored highest on the "emotional detachment" factor of the PCL-R. When study participants were regrouped based on their PCL-R factor scores, those who scored very high on both the emotional detachment and antisocial behavior factors showed blink inhibition for both pleasant and unpleasant pictures. Those with high antisocial scores but low detachment scores showed a normal pattern of startle inhibition for pleasant pictures and potentiation for unpleasant pictures. (See Figure 6.)

Subsequently, Patrick (1994) reported that--compared to nonpsychopaths and prisoners who scored high on the PCL-R antisocial factor only--psychopaths showed less startle potentiation during anticipation of an aversive event (i.e., loud noise blast) , and so did prisoners who were high on the PCL-R emotional detachment factor only. These results confirmed that reduced defensive reactivity (i.e., startle potentiation) is specifically related to the core emotional features of psychopathy. In another study, Mejia, Vanman, Dawson, Raine, and Lencz (1997) reported that volunteers from an employment agency who scored high on both factors of the PCL-R did not show startle reflex potentiation during unpleasant pictures, whereas volunteers who were high on the antisocial behavior factor did.

Patrick (1994) also reported correlations between the two PCL-R factors and temperament scales developed by Buss and Plomin (1975, 1984). Emotional detachment, controlling for antisocial behavior, was negatively related to self-ratings of Distress and Fear; antisocial behavior, controlling for emotional detachment, was related positively to Distress, Fear, Anger, and Impulsivity scales. Subsequently, Patrick (1995) examined relationships

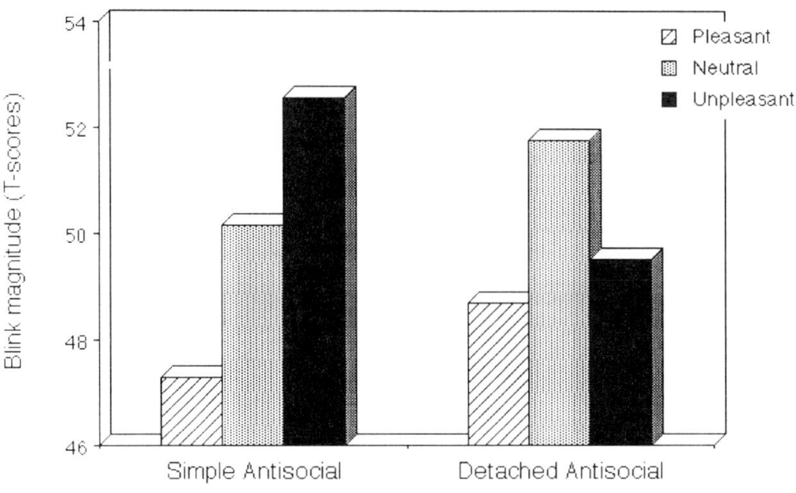

Figure 6. Mean startle blink magnitude (T-scores) during pleasant, neutral, and unpleasant pictures among male prisoners with high scores on the antisocial behavior factor but not the emotional detachment factor of the PCL-R ("simple antisocial"; n = 18), and among prisoners high on both PCL-R factors ("detached antisocial"; n = 17). Data are from an experiment by Patrick, Bradley, and Lang (1993).

between the PCL-R and Tellegen's (1982) Multidimensional Personality Questionnaire (MPQ), which measures 11 different temperament traits. Significant correlations were found between PCL-R emotional detachment scores and four MPQ trait scales--Social Potency (+), Achievement (+), Stress Reaction (-), and Traditionalism (-) (Patrick, 1995).. The antisocial behavior factor, on the other hand, was related to low Wellbeing, Achievement, and Control, and high Stress Reaction, Alienation, and Aggression.

8. EMOTION AND BEHAVIORAL (DIS)INHIBITION IN PSYCHOPATHY

The findings reviewed up to this point indicate that individuals who exhibit the core "emotional detachment" features of psychopathy have a higher threshold for defensive reactivity. Related to this, Lykken (1995) hypothesized that the basic abnormality in "primary" (true) psychopathy is low fearfulness. Individual differences in fearfulness exist because the defensive motivational system opposes approach behavior (Konorski, 1967; Lang, 1995), and because a weaker avoidance system can be adaptive in some environments. Specifically, when resources such as food or reproductive partners are in short supply, individuals with a high threshold for avoidance will enjoy a survival advantage. From this viewpoint, psychopaths are predatory individuals (Hare, 1993) who are specially adapted to survive in settings where resources are scarce and approach motivation must win out unless danger is close at hand.

In normal people, stimuli that are linked by past experience to pain or punishment automatically elicit a defensive action state that inhibits approach behavior. Behavior can be inhibited because a person is afraid of being punished themselves, or because the person recognizes that other people could be harmed by that behavior. In the case of psychopaths, the startle research data indicate that aversive stimuli must be more intense to elicit a defensive reaction that will interrupt goal-seeking behavior. That is, psychopaths react only to punishments that are immediate and personal; they are insensitive to the pain and discomfort of other people. As a result, the psychopath pursues selfish goals without regard to the immediate damage he does to others or the long-term trouble he causes himself.

Furthermore, the findings on emotion and temperament in criminal offenders suggest that different types of antisocial offenders may have different kinds of emotional processing deficits. "Primary" psychopathy appears to involve a basic deficit in fear reactivity—i.e., reduced defensive reactivity to aversive stimuli that are direct and explicit. However, antisocial offenders who are low on the emotional detachment factor of psychopathy show normal startle potentiation during exposure to aversive stimuli. Also, the temperament data indicate that antisocial behavior (controlling for emotional detachment) is related to higher trait anxiety and higher impulsivity. It was noted at the beginning of this paper that normal emotional processing involves higher cortical systems as well as subcortical motivation systems. Some forms of chronic antisocial deviance may result from deficits in higher brain systems that help to guide and inhibit behavior in situations where emotional stimuli are not explicit (LeDoux, 1995).

Consistent with this idea, there is substantial evidence that neuropsychological deficits, including abnormalities in prefrontal and temporal brain regions, are more common in antisocial individuals (Raine, 1993). Research on alcohol and emotional reactivity also supports the idea that behavioral deviance can result from disruptions in cognitive-emotional processing. Under the influence of alcohol, people are more likely to engage in deviant and reckless behaviors—including aggression, sexual risk-taking, and dangerous stunts. For many years, it was thought that alcohol directly suppressed the fear system that normally inhibits such behaviors. However, recent research using the startle probe technique indicates that alcohol affects fear response indirectly, by disrupting cognitive operations required to detect emotional stimuli that are subtle or that occur outside the immediate focus of attention (Curtin, Lang, Patrick, & Stritzke, 1998).

One hypothesis being addressed in our current work is that some aggressive antisocial offenders possess normal emotional response systems, but have difficulty inhibiting their behavior in complex situations because their cognitive processing systems are impaired. These individuals would be more similar to intoxicated persons than they would be to "primary" psychopaths.

9. EMOTION AND VIOLENT BEHAVIOR IN PSYCHOPATHS

Cleckley (1976) described psychopaths as lacking in strong emotions, including "violent rage", and his diagnostic criteria did not include any specific mention of aggressiveness. He stated that psychopaths do not usually commit major crimes of violence, and he concluded that "such tendencies should be regarded as the exception rather than the rule, perhaps, as a pathologic trait independent, to a considerable degree, of the other manifestations which we regard as fundamental" (p. 262).

However, empirical research has revealed a strong relationship between psychopathy and violent behavior in male criminal offenders (Patrick & Zempolich, 1998). Most published studies have reported a higher incidence and frequency of violent crime and aggressive behavior in high psychopathic individuals. Group differences tend to vary with crime type. Nonpsychopaths are more likely than psychopaths to be imprisoned for murder, which is usually a crime of passion committed against a known victim; psychopaths are more likely than nonpsychopaths to victimize strangers without killing them (Williamson, Hare, & Wong, 1987).

Psychopaths are also more likely to engage in aggressive and disruptive behavior in prison as a way to control others. Outside of prison, the violent crimes of psychopaths typically involve threats, physical force, and weapons. Psychopaths are also more likely than nonpsychopaths to victimize strangers in order to get money and other things from them (Williamson et al., 1987), and they are more likely to commit violent offenses after being released from prison, within a shorter period of time (Serin & Amos, 1995). These results indicate that psychopaths use aggression for purposes of manipulation and control. As further evidence of this, therapy outcome research indicates that treatment procedures designed to make offenders more sensitive to the feelings of other people actually <u>increase</u> the risk of violent reoffending among psychopaths (Harris, Rice, & Cormier, 1991).

There are a number of significant weaknesses in the literature on psychopathy and violent behavior (see Patrick & Zempolich, 1998). One is that relationships between psychopathy and aggression might arise because

PCL-R ratings are based on information about the offender that includes past acts of violence. A second limitation is that these studies have relied on official crime records, which usually underestimate the true frequency of offending. Furthermore, not all of these studies classified violent crimes into different subtypes, and those that did used a crude classification approach based on official crime codes. As a result, almost no firm evidence exists concerning the reasons (motives) for violent offending in psychopaths.

However, the correlations that have been reported between the PCL-R and personality trait measures provide a way to think about connections between psychopathy and aggressive behavior. The contrasting relationships between the two psychopathy factors and MPQ personality traits are especially interesting. Antisocial behavior is related to higher stress, aggression, and impulsiveness. This suggests that the connection between the PCL-R and defensive aggression (also known as "angry" or "reactive" aggression; Buss, 1961, and Dodge, 1991) is mediated by the antisocial behavior factor. On the other hand, PCL-R emotional detachment, after controlling for antisocial behavior, is related to high social dominance and ambition, as well as low anxiety. This indicates that aggression in the "true" (Cleckley) psychopath is more likely to be goal-directed (i.e., "instrumental" or "proactive"; Buss [1961], Dodge [1991]) than defensive.

Patrick, Zempolich, and Levenston (1997) examined relationships between the two PCL-R factors and different forms of aggressive behavior. Their findings were generally consistent with the hypotheses mentioned above. The antisocial behavior factor of the PCL-R was related to several different measures of impulsive, angry aggression: assault offenses; aggressive behaviors as a child (i.e., bullying or threatening other children; starting fights; deliberately hurting animals or people; sexually abusive behavior); reported frequency of fights as an adult; and physically abuse of spouse or partner. The emotional detachment factor was related more to planned, instrumental aggression (i.e. possession and use of weapons; see Harpur & Hare, 1991). Figure 7 depicts relationships between PCL-R ratings of prisoners and frequency scores for four violent crime categories.

10. SUMMARY AND CONCLUSIONS

This paper has reviewed findings concerning emotion, temperament, and aggressive behavior in psychopathic individuals. Studies of emotion using the startle-probe technique and of temperament using the MPQ indicate that the core emotional detachment factor of psychopathy is related to a weak defensive activation system and to traits of high dominance and low anxiousness. Studies of aggression and psychopathy indicate that psychopathic individuals are more likely than nonpsychopaths to commit violent crimes of a forceful nature in order to achieve immediate goals.

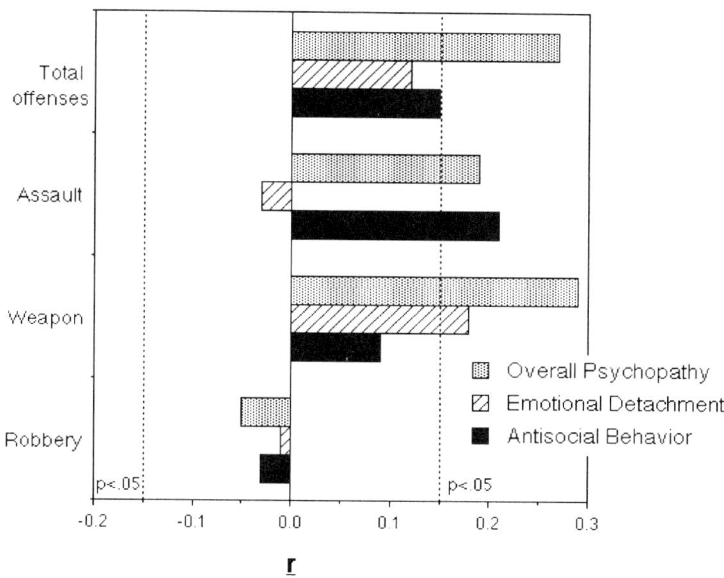

Figure 7. Relationships between ratings of incarcerated criminal offenders (N = 214) on the two PCL-R factors and number of violent offenses listed in criminal records. Correlations are presented for all violence crimes combined, and for specific offenses with the highest base rates (assault, weapons-related, and robbery).

Thus, the picture that emerges of the true psychopath is that of a predatory individual who uses violence to intimidate others and to achieve selfish aims.

Angry, reactive aggression is more likely to be committed by antisocial individuals who do not exhibit the emotional detachment of the true psychopath. In these individuals, violent behavior is more likely to result from deficits in cognitive functions that normally work together with the primary emotion systems. Drugs like alcohol that disrupt emotional processing by impairing attention and memory may provide a useful experimental method for examining this type of antisocial aggression (Patrick & Lang, 1999).

REFERENCES

American Psychiatric Association. (1994): *Diagnostic and statistical manual of mental disorders* (4th ed.), Washington, DC, Author.

Anthony, B. J. & Graham, F. K. (1985): "Blink reflex modification by selective attention: Evidence for the modulation of 'automatic' processing", *Biological Psychology*, 20, pp. 43-59.

Arnett, P. A. (1997): "Autonomic responsivity in psychopaths: A critical review and theoretical proposal". *Clinical Psychology Review*, 17, pp. 903-936.

Buss, A. (1961): *The psychology of aggression*, New York, Wiley.

Buss, A. H. & Plomin, R. (1975): *A temperament theory of personality development*, New York, Wiley.

Buss, A. H. & Plomin, R. (1984): *Temperament: Early developing personality traits*, Hillsdale, NJ, Erlbaum.

Christianson, S-Å; Forth, A. E.; Hare, R. D.; Strachan, C.; Lidberg, L. & Thorell, L-H. (1996): "Remembering details of emotional events: A comparison between psychopathic and nonpsychopathic offenders", *Personality and Individual Differences*, 20, pp. 437-443.

Cleckley, H. (1976): *The mask of sanity* (5th ed.), St. Louis, MO, Mosby.

Curtin, J. J.; Lang, A. R.; Patrick, C. J. & Stritzke, W. G. K. (1998): "Alcohol and fear-potentiated startle: The role of distraction in the stress-reducing effects of intoxication", *Journal of Abnormal Psychology*, 107, pp. 545-555.

Cuthbert, B. N.; Bradley, M. M. & Lang, P. J. (1996): "Probing picture perception: Activation and emotion", *Psychophysiology*, 33, pp. 103-111.

Davis, M. (1979): "Diazepam and flurazepam: Effects on conditioned fear as measured with the potentiated startle paradigm", *Psychopharmacology*, 62, pp. 1-7.

Davis, M. (1989): "Neural systems involved in fear-potentiated startle", in M. Davis, B. L. Jacobs & R.I. Schoenfeld (Eds.), *Annals of the New York Academy of Sciences*, vol. 563: Modulation of defined neural vertebrate circuits. pp. 165-183, New York, Author.

Dodge, K. A. (1991): "The structure and function of reactive and proactive aggression", in D. J. Pepler & K. H. Rubin (Eds.), *The development and treatment of childhood aggression*, Hillsdale, NJ, Erlbaum.

Ekman, P. (1992): "An argument for basic emotions", *Cognition and Emotion*, 6, pp. 169-200.

Fanselow, M. S. (1994): "Neural organization of the defensive behavior system responsible for fear", *Psychonomic Bulletin and Review*, 1, pp. 429-438.

Fowles, D. C. (1980): "The three arousal model: Implications of Gray's two-factor learning theory for heart rate, electrodermal activity, and psychopathy", *Psychophysiology*, 17, pp. 87-104.

Gray, J. A. (1987): *The psychology of fear and stress* (2nd ed.), Cambridge, University of Cambridge Press.

Greenwald, M. K.; Cook, E.W. & Lang, P. J. (1989): "Affective judgment and psychophysiological response: Dimensional covariation in the evaluation of pictorial stimuli", *Journal of Psychophysiology*, 3, pp. 51-64.

Hare, R. D. (1970): *Psychopathy: Theory and research*, New York, Wiley.

Hare, R. D. (1978): "Electrodermal and cardiovascular correlates of psychopathy", in R. D. Hare & D. Schalling (Eds.), *Psychopathic behavior: Approaches to research*, Chichester, Wiley.

Hare, R. D. (1980): "A research scale for the assessment of psychopathy in criminal populations", *Personality and Individual Differences*, 1, pp. 111-119.

Hare, R. D. (1991): *The Hare Psychopathy Checklist-Revised*, Toronto, Multi-Health Systems.

Hare, R. D. (1993): *Without conscience: The disturbing world of the psychopaths among us*, New York, Pocket Books.

Harpur, T. J.; Hakstian, A. R. & Hare, R. D. (1988): "Factor structure of the psychopathy checklist", *Journal of Consulting and Clinical Psychology*, 56, pp. 741-747.

Harpur, T. J. & Hare, R. D. (August 1991): *Psychopathy and violent behavior: Two factors are better than one*, Paper presented at the 99 Annual Meeting of the American Psychological Association, San Francisco, CA.

Harpur, T. J.; Hare, R. D. & Hakstian, A. R. (1989): "Two-factor conceptualization of psychopathy: Construct validity and assessment implications", *Psychological Assessment: A Journal of Consulting and Clinical Psychology*, 1, pp. 6-17.

Hebb, D. O. (1955): "Drives and the C.N.S. (conceptual nervous system)", *Psychological Review*, 62, pp. 243-254.

Izard, C. E. (1993): "Four systems for emotion activation: Cognitive and noncognitive processes", *Psychological Review*, 100, pp. 68-90.

Jutai, J. W. & Hare, R. D. (1983): "Psychopathy and selective attention during performance of a complex perceptual-motor task", *Psychophysiology*, 20, pp. 146-151.

Konorski, J. (1967): *Integrative activity of the brain: An interdisciplinary approach*, Chicago, University of Chicago Press.

Kosson, D. S. (1996): "Psychopathy and dual-task performance under focusing conditions", *Journal of Abnormal Psychology*, 105, pp. 391-400.

Kosson, D. S. (1998): "Divided visual attention in psychopathic and nonpsychopathic offenders", *Personality and Individual Differences*, 24, pp. 373-391.

Kosson, D. S. & Harpur, T. J. (1997): "Attention functioning and psychopathic individuals: Current evidence and developmental implications", in J. A. Burack & J. T. Enns (Eds.), *Attention, development, and psychopathology*, New York, Guilford Press.

Kosson, D. S. & Newman, J. P. (1986): "Psychopathy and allocation of attentional capacity in a divided-attention situation", *Journal of Abnormal Psychology*, 95, pp. 257-263.

Lang, P. J. (1994): "The motivational organization of emotion: Affect-reflex connections", in S. Van Goozen, N. E. Van de Poll & J. A. Sergeant (Eds)., *The emotions: Essays on emotion theory*, Hillsdale, NJ, Lawrence Erlbaum.

Lang, P. J. (1995): "The emotion probe: Studies of motivation and attention", *American Psychologist*, 50, pp. 372-385.

Lang, P. J.; Bradley, M. M. & Cuthbert, B. N. (1990): "Emotion, attention, and the startle reflex", *Psychological Review*, 97, pp. 377-398.

Lang, P. J.; Bradley, M. M. & Cuthbert, B. N. (1997): "Motivated attention: Affect, activation, and action", in P. J. Lang, R. F. Simons & M. T. Balaban (Eds.), *Attention and orienting: Sensory and motivational processes*, Mahwah, NJ, Lawrence Erlbaum Associates, Inc.

Lazarus, R. (1982): "Thoughts on the relations between emotion and cognition". *American Psychologist* , 37, pp. 1019-1024.

Lazarus, R. (1984): "On the primacy of cognition", *American Psychologist*, 39, pp. 124-129.

LeDoux, J. E. (1995): "Emotion: Clues from the brain", *Annual Review of Psychology*, 46, pp. 209-235.

Levenston, G. K. & Patrick, C. J. (1995): "Probing the time course of picture processing: Emotional valence and stimulus content", *Psychophysiology*, 32, p. S50.

Levenston, G. K.; Patrick, C. J.; Bradley, M. M. & Lang, P. J. (in press): "The psychopath as observer: Emotion and attention in picture processing", *Journal of Abnormal Psychology*.

Lindsley, D. B. (1951): "Emotions", in S. S. Stevens (Ed.), *Handbook of experimental psychology*, New York, Wiley.

Lykken, D. T. (1957): "A study of anxiety in the sociopathic personality", *Journal of Abnormal and Clinical Psychology*, 55, pp. 6-10.

Lykken, D. T. (1995): *The antisocial personalities*, Hillsdale, NJ, Erlbaum.

Öhman, A. (1993): "Fear and anxiety as emotional phenomena: Clinical phenomenology, evolutionary perspectives, and information processing mechanisms", in M. Lewis & J. M. Haviland (Eds.), *Handbook of emotions* pp. 511-536, New York, Guilford.

MacLean, P. D. (1958): "Contrasting functions of limbic and neocortical systems of the brain and their relevance to psychophysiological aspects of medicine", *American Journal of Medicine*, 25, pp. 611-626.

Mejia, V. Y.; Vanman, E. J.; Dawson, M. E.; Raine, A. & Lencz, T. (1997): "An examination of affective modulation, psychopathy, and negative schizotypy in a nonincarcerated sample", *Psychophysiology*, 34, p S63.

Newman, J. P. & Wallace, J. F. (1993): "Psychopathy and Cognition", in P. C. Kendall & K. S. Dobson (Eds.), *Psychopathology and cognition*, pp. 293-349. New York, Academic Press.

Newman, J. P.; Schmitt, W. A. & Voss, W. D. (1997): "The impact of motivationally neutral cues on psychopathic individuals: Assessing the generality of the response modulation hypothesis", *Journal of Abnormal Psychology*, 106, pp. 563-575.

Papez, J. W. (1937): "A proposed mechanism of emotion", *Archives of Neurology and Psychiatry*, 38, pp. 725-743.

Patrick, C. J. (in press): "Stress reactivity: Biobehavioral insights", in K. D. Craig, R. J. McMahon & K. S. Dobson (Eds.), *Stress: Vulnerability and resilience*, New York, Sage.

Patrick, C. J. (Autumn 1995): "Emotion and temperament in psychopathy", *Clinical Science*, pp. 5-8.

Patrick, C. J. (1994): "Emotion and psychopathy: Startling new insights", *Psychophysiology*, 31, pp. 319-330.

Patrick, C. J.; Berthot, B. D. & Moore, J. D. (1996): "Diazepam blocks fear-potentiated startle in humans", *Journal of Abnormal Psychology*, 105, pp. 89-96.

Patrick, C. J.; Bradley, M. M. & Lang, P. J. (1993): "Emotion in the criminal psychopath: Startle reflex modulation", *Journal of Abnormal Psychology*, 102, pp. 82-92.

Patrick, C. J.; Cuthbert, B. N. & Lang, P. J. (1994): "Emotion in the criminal psychopath: Fear image processing", *Journal of Abnormal Psychology*, 103, pp. 523-534.

Patrick, C. J. & Lang, A. R. (1999): "Psychopathic traits and intoxicated states: Affective concomitants and conceptual links", in M. Dawson & A. Schell (Eds.), *Startle modification: Implications for clinical science, cognitive science, and neuroscience*, New York, Cambridge University Press.

Patrick, C. J. & Zempolich, K. A. (1998): "Emotion and aggression in the psychopathic personality", *Aggression and Violent Behavior*, 3, pp. 303-338.

Patrick, C. J.; Zempolich, K. A. & Levenston, G. K. (1997): "Emotionality and violent behavior in psychopaths: A biosocial analysis", in A. Raine, D. Farrington, P. Brennan & S. A. Mednick (Eds.), *The biosocial bases of violence*, New York, Plenum.

Plutchik, R. (1984): "Emotions: A general psychoevolutionary theory", in K. Scherer & P. Ekman (Eds.), *Approaches to emotion*, Hillsdale, NJ, Erlbaum.

Raine, A. (1993): *The psychopathology of crime*, San Diego, Academic Press.

Rice, M. E.; Harris, G. T. & Cormier, C.A. (1992): "An evaluation of a maximum security therapeutic community for psychopaths and other mentally disordered offenders", *Law and Human Behavior*, 16, pp. 399-412.

Russell, J. A. & Mehrabian, A. (1977): "Evidence for a three-factor theory of emotions", *Journal of Research in Personality*, 11, pp. 273-294.

Schachter, S. (1964): "The interaction of cognitive and physiological determinants of emotional state", in L. Berkowitz (Ed.), *Advances in experimental social psychology* (vol. 1), New York, Academic Press.

Schneirla, T. C. (1959): "An evolutionary and developmental theory of biphasic processes underlying approach and withdrawal", in *Nebraska Symposium on Motivation: 1959*, Lincoln, University of Nebraska Press.

Serin, R. C. & Amos, N. L. (1995): "The role of psychopathy in the assessment of dangerousness", *International Journal of Law and Psychiatry*, 18, pp. 231-238.

Smith, S. S. & Newman, J. P. (1990): "Alcohol and drug abuse-dependence disorders in psychopathic and nonpsychopathic criminal offenders", *Journal of Abnormal Psychology*, 99, pp. 430-439.

Stritzke, W. G. K.; Lang, A. R. & Patrick, C. J. (1996): "Beyond stress and arousal: A reconceptualization of alcohol-emotion relations with special reference to psychophysiological methods", *Psychological Bulletin*, 120, pp. 376-395.

Tellegen, A. (1982): *Brief manual for the Multidimensional Personality Questionnaire*, (unpublished manuscript), University of Minnesota.

Williamson, S.; Hare, R. D. & Wong, S. (1987): "Violence: criminal psychopaths and their victims", *Canadian Journal of Behavioral Science*, 19, pp. 454-462.

Williamson, S.; Harpur, T. J. & Hare, R. D. (1991): "Abnormal processing of affective words by psychopaths", *Psychophysiology*, 28, pp. 260-273.

Zajonc, R. B. (1980): "Feeling and thinking: Preferences need no inferences", *American Psychologist*, 35, pp. 151-175.

Zajonc, R. B. (1984): "On the primacy of affect", *American Psychologist*, 39, pp. 117-123.

Chapter 4

NEUROBIOLOGY OF THE PSYCHOPATH

James Santiago Grisolía
Section of Neurology, Scripps-Mercy Hospital, San Diego, California

1. INTRODUCTION

Books, movies and articles about serial killers, usually psychopathic, have become regular staples of modern culture. Our fascination with psychopaths and serial killers seems to well up from a deep, dark place within us, a place that yearns for an absence of constraints, that longs for unfettered domination of others. We are afraid of that dark, glittering place inside us, so that the wise detective, the hunt for justice, the comforting end to the chase satisfies us, leaving us in control again. An obsessive story of violence and control repeats itself in endless versions, a deep mythos of our times.

Where is that dark place, and why does its siren song keep calling us? Within each of us lies a hard, reptilian core of need. Neurophysiology places that core of primal needs in our brainstem and limbic system; evolution and our individual development bury those needs under many layers of inhibition, of learned responses, of conditioned stimuli taking the place of primary stimuli. This process of conditioning, of restraining that primitive core breaks down in the psychopath, leading to an impoverished internal emotional life and an inability to empathize with others. It also leads to special kinds of violence and aggressive behavior, distinct from the majority of aggressors or convicted felons.

When biologists speak about behavior, they focus on general principles. In an experiment on aggression in rats, one speaks of the interplay of aggression centers with each other, other brain areas and external factors (drugs, brain injury, emotional deprivation, other rats, cats or mice) without distinguishing between one rat and another in its reactions and behavior. Speaking of humans, biologically-oriented scientists continue to focus on general principles of physiology and behavior, while clinicians—psychologists, neurologists and psychiatrists—are more interested in individual differences. Clinicians think in terms of *syndromes*, or clusters of clinical characteristics.

Violence and Psychopathy, edited by Raine & Sanmartin,
Kluwer Academic/Plenum Publishers, New York, 2001.

In reality, both perspectives are essential. On one hand, any group of people exposed to certain biological or environmental factors will have a higher probability of violent action. On the other hand, each person is an individual, the unique result of multiple, complex factors, so that one abused individual may grow up resolving to break the cycle of violence while another continues to abuse his children or wife. The great variability in human behavior requires distinctions, so that speaking of clinical syndromes conveniently expresses the similarities and differences between some people and others.

Importantly, recognizing syndromic differences in behavior does not immediately explain causation. Everyone can tell the difference between depression and manic elation, although they might not use the clinical words for these two syndromes. It will take the biological skills of neuropharmacology, neurophysiology, genetics and other specialties to fully understand the causes of these syndromes. The clinical and biological approaches each enrich the other. The clinician finds the differences; the biologist attempts to explain them.

Within the study of violent individuals, it is convenient to distinguish psychopaths from other violent individuals as a separate syndrome. As well outlined in the chapter by Hare (this volume), psychopaths have distinct attitudes, behaviors, types of violence, and risk for repeat crimes. Psychopaths have a peculiar, striking affect disorder—superficial pleasantness, facile lying, the capacity to kill in cold blood. In some sense, *cold blood* best captures what is most characteristic about the psychopath.

Trying to describe what separates the psychopath from other prisoners or patients is difficult. The terms antisocial personality and psychopathy illustrate the distinction between statistical/demographic and clinical approaches to defining this group of people. The varying definitions of antisocial personality focus on statistical counting of crimes and violent acts. The definition of psychopathy, as embodied in the PCL-R and related test instruments developed by Hare and his cohorts, includes the clinical perspective of recognizing the importance of the very distinctive psychopathic personality, in addition to the antisocial acts themselves. A key contribution of Dr Hare has been to clarify the importance of the psychopath's personality and his relation to other persons.

2. THE PSYCHOBIOLOGY OF VIOLENCE

We can begin by speaking of violence from a more general, biologic perspective, later applying these findings to the psychopath. The visceral reactions of a frightened or angry person—the leap of the pulse, the cold sweat, the enlarged pupils—are controlled by the autonomic nervous system. The autonomic nervous system is regulated by certain nuclei in the hypothalamus and by the limbic system, including its structures and connections within the temporal lobe (especially the amygdala) and with the medial and orbital surfaces of the frontal lobes. The same centers control other aspects of emotion, as well, so that our internal experience of an emotion, such as anger, is inextricably bound to external signs—facial expression, rising blood pressure and pulse, etc.

Unfortunately, the frontal and temporal lobes are highly susceptible to injury, including from head trauma, child abuse, etc, so that many persons receive injuries that affect the control of their emotional centers, leading them to uncontrolled emotions and violent behavior. For the most part these individuals are emotionally disinhibited, so that they get frustrated more easily by small provocations, then are incapable of controlling their aggressive actions. Large-scale studies of abused children show that only certain children will in turn adopt aggressive or abusive strategies themselves. The children that become aggressive themselves have developed defective social programming skills, either from the abuse experience itself or from some other aspect of the environment (Dodge, 1993).

The classic studies of Pincus and colleagues demonstrate that the behavioral effects of acquired brain lesions (usually diffuse or predominantly frontotemporal) can interact with an abusive environment. Persons with brain lesions, if they are abused as children, can sometimes adopt a paranoid attitude and learn from their abusers that violence is an efficient method for controlling others, becoming violent criminals (Lewis et al., 1987; Blake et al., 1995).

Various personality traits may have a genetic component, including aggression. Twin studies may help define the genetic component in many aspects of behavior. Identical (monozygotic, or MZ) twins share 100% of their genetic material, while fraternal (dizygotic, or DZ) twins share about 50% of their genome, like any other pair of siblings. If a predisposition to violence exists on a genetic basis identical twins would agree on this trait more often than fraternal twins. Additionally, studies of siblings versus step-siblings also assist in separating genetic effects from the effects of a shared environment.

A simple means of measuring violent conduct uses a parent questionnaire, counting details such as frequency of aggressive behaviors against other children, frequency of arguments with parents, cruelty, etc. A study by this technique found correlations of .83 in MZ twins and .62 in DZ twins, indicating a genetic contribution of some 42% to the overall variation in this behavior (Cadoret et al., 1997). Another twin study found correlation of .78 for MZ and .31 for DZ (Ghodesian-Carpey & Baker, 1987). Among adopted children, siblings sharing the same biologic parents showed higher correlations regarding aggressive behaviors than siblings with different biologic parents (Van der Oord et al., 1994). A very exhaustive study of 720 adolescents between 10 and 18 years of age, included twins and siblings sharing both, one or no biologic parents. These teens were rated for aggressive behaviors by independent observers during arguments with their parents, with the result that approximately 28% of variation in aggression could be explained by genetic factors (Reiss et al., 1994).

Arrests and convictions for violent offenses provide a different measure of violent behavior, carrying the obvious advantage of real-world relevance. Potential disadvantages include socioeconomic influences, including ethnicity of offenders, available resources for legal defense, access to illegal activities, etc. In a group of juvenile offenders, 30% of variability in criminal aggression was explained genetically (DiLalla & Gottesman, 1989). In a group of 4,997 Danish men, (from a society which is relatively homogenous ethnically, socially, etc), some 50% of variability in crimes against persons was explained by genetic factors and 67% of variability in crimes against property (Cloninger & Gottesman, 1987).

Our understanding of brain function is still too limited to specifically identify the diverse genes that influence behavior, but already several single gene defects have been characterized which increase aggressive behavior, including defects in nitric oxide synthetase (Nelson et al., 1995), in MAO synthetase A (Cases et al., 1995), and the Lesch-Nyhan syndrome (Anderson & Ernst, 1994). Although none of these defects would explain aggressive behaviors in a clinically normal population, they nevertheless demonstrate that, at least under some environmental and biological conditions, genetic abnormalities can lead to aggressive behavior. Brain centers involved in emotional control (frontal/temporal lobes, limbic system, autonomic nervous system) are the most promising functional zones for genetic research relevant to aggressive behavior. Certain neurotransmitter systems, especially serotonin (to a lesser extent catecholaminergic neurons), play important roles in regulation of affective behaviors including aggression; potential genetic polymorphism in function of these systems might also explain much of human aggression (Eichelman & Hartwig, 1997).

Biologic systems never function independently of their environments, and many social factors influence violent behaviors by interacting with unstable or predisposed biological systems. Important environmental factors include exposure to media violence (Wilson et al., 1997), availability of firearms (Cook & Cole, 1996), economic inequality within society (Pampel & Gartner, 1995), and perinatal/prenatal complications (Kandel, 1992).

3. PSYCHOBIOLOGY OF THE PSYCHOPATH

When we attempt to focus on the psychopath, we find various difficulties. Most large-scale studies are based on behaviors (childhood aggression, criminal arrests, etc) with only rare reference to the specific diagnosis of the violent subjects. This point is crucial, as the majority of aggressive individuals or even convicted criminals are not psychopaths, even though committing criminal acts is needed to fulfill definitions for either antisocial personality or psychopathy. For example, in various populations of young U.S. males, the frequency of non-traffic convictions reaches 25% to 47%, while only 3% of the same demographic groups qualify for the diagnosis of antisocial personality (Farrington, 1986). Even in prison populations, the majority do not qualify for definitions of antisocial personality or psychopathy (Hart & Hare, 1989).

Psychopathy is defined by repeated antisocial acts, along with the abnormal affect and the self-report of bizarre or absent internal emotional experience described by Hare and others. Crucially, this affect disturbance includes an inability to understand the actual or possible victim as having emotions, making cold-blooded, instrumental crimes appear not only possible but even inconsequential. Acquired lesions (trauma, brain tumors, etc) of frontal and temporal lobe limbic structures can result in antisocial behavior (crimes, domestic abuse, etc), but these are usually impulsive, irritative acts without the peculiar cold-blooded affect of classic psychopathy Grisolía, 1997). Nevertheless, psychopaths clearly show abnormal processing of emotionally-charged information, as well discussed by Patrick in this volume. This strongly implies that they do have abnormalities in limbic centers, including frontal and temporal lobe structures. How are they different from other people with frontal and/or temporal lobe damage?

Recently, Damasio et al have published anecdotal cases of lesions to the inferior and medial surfaces of frontal lobe acquired very early in life, associated with an apparent psychopathic affective disturbance (Anderson et al., 1999). This suggests that intact frontomedial systems may be required in early life to develop functioning cognitive models of personal emotional experience, as well as the ability to project this emotional model outside oneself onto other people. A pathbreaking study by Raine and colleagues used quantitative MRI in a group of psychopaths to demonstrate reduced gray matter and increased white matter in frontal lobe (Raine et al., 2000). Perhaps the majority of psychopaths have some sort of early life disruption that makes their frontal lobes develop differently. Decreased gray matter could be due to any kind of damage causing atrophy, but the *increase* in white matter suggests defective pruning, a hallmark of changes in development of neural circuitry in the growing brain.

Epidemiologic studies have long demonstrated an association of adverse prenatal and perinatal complications with psychopathy and/or antisocial behavior in the offspring (Kandel, 1992). However, it has been difficult to tease apart genetic and other environmental effects from the more immediate effects of prenatal disturbance, because of the strong correlations between prenatal/perinatal complications, socioeconomic status, and drug/alcohol dependencies. A recent analysis of children born during the Great Famine in the Netherlands during WWII now demonstrates that nutritional deprivation during the first or second trimester increases the risk of antisocial behavior in offspring, independent of other environmental or genetic factors (Neugebauer et al., 1999). This study is especially convincing, because it involved an ethnically and socially homogenous society which was subjected to severe malnutrition due to external circumstances, with relative preservation of other social structures.

Malnutrition has significant effects on brain growth and development, which have been best studied postnatally, but may occur in modified form prenatally as well (Pollitt et al., 1995). Other, simpler examples are known where gene expression may be differentially affected by maternal or intra-uterine environmental factors (Adams et al., 1997). This fits with the MRI data on psychopaths, who may respond to prenatal or early life adversity through changes in frontal lobe development and subsequent behavior (this could also interact with other potential factors, such as genetic predisposition). Already, studies of adopted children suggest that biological offspring of antisocial parents are less likely to become antisocial themselves if raised in a good home than in a bad home (Cadoret et al., 1995).

Taken together, these data support the intriguing possibility that psychopathy could be part of a range of evolved behavioral responses to environmental factors. For a child born into a time of maternal hardship, more directly self-oriented behavior may be more survival-oriented, while in a time of greater plenty, more altruistic, mutually cooperative behavior might be more adaptive. This hypothesis has the superficial ring of plausibility, but obviously requires much more thought and testing.

Evolutionary explanations for behavior smuggle teleology into scientific discussion and therefore must be regarded with extreme caution. However, this idea yields several interesting implications. Firstly, the possibility that psychopathy may be adaptive in some extreme environments is disturbing and clearly requires further assessment, possibly by cross-cultural studies. Secondly, the concept that psychopathy might represent the extreme end of a spectrum of altruistic behavior refocuses interest on so-called "adaptive psychopaths" and/or individuals with mild to moderate elevations on the PCL-R or similar instruments for rating psychopathy, two groups which may or may not be identical (Forth et al., 1996). Up until now, most clinical and investigative work has understandably focussed on prison and other criminalized populations of psychopaths.

Within evolutionary biology, altruistic behavior remains an unresolved issue, generating competing theories on its adaptive value for the individual versus for the social unit (Bradley, 1999). Further study of high-functioning psychopaths, and/or study of individuals with moderate psychopathy scores, may shed light on this issue. This hypothesis may provide additional insight into genetic mechanisms of behavior and facilitate a search for animal models of psychopathy. Lastly, the idea that prenatal and early-life factors may impact frontal and/or limbic development and long-term criminality should serve as a fresh stimulus for the prevention of brain dysfunction in at-risk populations.

4. CONCLUSION

We can reliably differentiate the psychopath from other criminal or psychiatric patients. In general, we know that brainstem centers control our primal needs, with inhibition and modification by limbic centers in the temporal and frontal lobes of the brain. These limbic centers are fragile and can be disrupted by many processes. Brain injuries acquired during life usually result in irritative, impulsive violence. Emerging evidence suggests that frontal lobe disruption occurring prenatally or very early in childhood may cause psychopathy (resulting in instrumental, or "cold-blooded" violence instead of impulsive violence) by preventing the formation of internal emotional models so the individual cannot project those emotional models onto others. By growing up without internal meanings for emotions, the psychopath cannot understand that others can be hurt, offended, suffer, etc.

The Great Famine in Holland showed that malnutrition during the first 2 trimesters of pregnancy causes increased antisocial behavior and an MRI study of American psychopaths found abnormal brain development in the frontal lobes. Malnutrition and other adverse prenatal experiences appear to contribute to psychopathy, perhaps by adaptive alteration of frontal lobe development; this offers hope for prevention and potential future research directions.

Potentially important environmental prevention factors include such basics as prenatal nutrition and medical care, improved parent-child relations, maternal drug and alcohol use, etc. For the foreseeable future, it will remain easier, cheaper and more humane to optimize the environment of pregnant women and young children than to alter biology.

The psychopathic killer continues to obsess our culture. His demonic urges echo our own restless energy, still whirring uneasily in our brainstems; under other circumstances, his cold impulses might be ours. In our world of control and inhibition, the fantasy of moving unseen, all powerful, able to defeat police and all civil authority, appeals to us deeply, yet the final taming of the psychopath leaves us slaked. Lacking empathy or any developed emotional life, the psychopath may be said to be less human than the rest of us; yet we still respond with a horrified fascination to his presence, perhaps the rodent wavering before the lunge of the snake. Knowing, of course, that we each carry the serpent's hunger and guile within our rodent hearts.

REFERENCES

Adams, S. H.; Alho, C. S.; Asins, G. et al. (1997): "Gene expression of mitochondrial 3-hydroxy-3-methylglutaryl-CoA synthase in a ketogenic mammal: Effect of starvation during the neonatal period of the piglet", *Biochemical Journal*, 324 (1), pp. 65-73.

Anderson, L. T. & Ernst, M. (1994): "Self-injury in Lesch-Nyhan disease", *Journal Autism Developmental Disabilities*, 24 (1), pp. 67-81.

Anderson, S. W.; Bechara, A.; Damasio, H.; Travel, D. & Damasio, A. R. (1999): "Impairment of social and moral behavior related to early damage in human prefrontal cortex", *Nature Neuroscience*, 2 (11), pp. 1032-7.

Blake, P. Y.; Pincus, J. H. & Buckner, C. (1995): "Neurologic abnormalities in murderers", *Neurology*, 45, pp. 1641-1647.

Bradley, B. J. (1999): "Levels of selection, altruism and primate behavior", *Quarterly Review of Biology*, 74 (2), pp. 171-94.

Cadoret, R. J.; Leve, L. D. & Devor, E. (1997): "Genetics of violent behaviors", *Psychiatric Clinics of North America*, 20, pp. 301-321.

Cadoret, R. J.; Troughton, E.; Bagford, J. et al. (1995): "Genetic-environmental interaction in the genesis of aggressivity and conduct disorders", *Archives General Psychiatry*, 52, pp. 916-919.

Cases, O. et al. (1995): "Aggressive behavior and altered amounts of brain serotonin and norepinephrine in mice lacking MAOA", *Science*, 268, pp. 1763-1766.

Cloninger, D. R. & Gottesman, I. I. (1987): "Genetic and environmental factors in antisocial behavior disorders", in S. A. Mednick (ed.), *The Causes of Crime: New Biological Approaches*, New York, Cambridge Univ., pp. 92-109.

Cook, P. J. & Cole, T. B. (1996): "Strategic thinking about gun markets and violence", *JAMA*, 275, pp. 1765-67.

DiLalla, L. F. & Gottesman, I. I. (1989): "Heterogeneity of causes for delinquency and criminality", *Developmental Psychopathology*, 1, pp. 339-347.

Dodge, K. A. (1993): "Studying mechanisms in the cycle of violence", in C. Thompson & P. Cowen (eds), *Violence: Basic and Clinical Science*, London, Butterworth, pp. 19-34.

Eichelman, B. & Hartwig, A. (1997): "Classification of violent syndromes", in J. Grisolía, J. Sanmartin et al. (eds), *Violence: From Biology to Society*, Amsterdam, Elsevier, pp. 25-34.

Farrington, D. P. (1986): "Age and crime", in M. Towry & N. Morris (eds), *Crime and Justice: An Annual Review of Research*, Vol 7, Chicago, University of Chicago.

Forth, A. E.; Brown, S. L.; Hart, S. D. & Hare, R. D. (1996): "The assessment of psychopathy in male and female noncriminals: Reliability and validity", *Personality and Individual Differences*, 20, pp. 531-543.

Ghodesian-Carpey, J. & Baker, L. A. (1987): "Genetic and environmental influences on aggression in 4- to 7-year old twins", *Aggression and Behavior*, 13, pp. 173-177.

Grisolía, J. (1997): "Temporal lobe mechanisms and violence", in J. Grisolía, J. Sanmartín et al. (eds), *Violence: From Biology to Society*, Amsterdam, Elsevier, pp. 43-52.

Hart, S.D. & Hare, R. D. (1989): "Discriminant validity of the Psychopathy Checklist in a forensic psychiatric population", *Psychology Assessments*, 1, pp. 211-218.

Kandel, E (1992): "Biology, violence and antisocial personality", *Journal Forensic Science*, 37, pp. 912-918.

Lewis, D. O.; Pincus, J. H.; Lovely, R. et al. (1987): "Biopsychosocial characteristics of matched samples of delinquents and non-delinquents", *Journal of American Academy Child and Adolescent Psychiatry*, 26, pp. 744-752.

Nelson, R. J. et al. (1995): "Behavioral abnormalities in male mice lacking neuronal nitric oxide synthase", *Nature*, 378, 383-386.

Neugebauer, R.; Hoek, W. & Susser, E. (1999): "Prenatal exposure to wartime famine and development of antisocial personality disorder in early adulthood", *JAMA*, 282, pp. 455-462.

Pampel, F. C. & Gartner, R. (1995): "Age structure, sociopolitical institutions and national homicide rates", *European Sociology Review*, 11, pp. 243-260.

Pollitt, E.; Gorman, K. S.; Engle, P. I. et al. (1995): "Nutrition in early life and the fulfillment of intellectual potential", *Journal of Nutrition*, 125 (Suppl. 4), pp. 1111S-1118S.

Raine, A.; Lencz, T.; Behrle, S.; LaCasse, L. & Colletti, P. (2000): "Reduced prefrontal gray volume and reduced autonomic activity in antisocial personality disorder", *Archives General Psychiatry*, 57 (2), pp. 119-27.

Reiss, D.; Plomin, R.; Hetherington, E. M. et al. (1994): "The separate worlds of teenage siblings: An introduction to the study of the nonshared environment and adolescent development", in E. M. Hetherington (ed.), *Separate Social Worlds of Siblings: Importance of Nonshared Environment on Development*, Hillsdale, Erlbaum, pp. 63-110.

Van der Oord, E. J.; Boomsma, D. I. & Verhulst, F. C. (1994): "A study of problem behaviors in 10- to 15-year old biologically related and unrelated international adoptees", *Behavioral Genetics*, 24, pp. 193-205.

Wilson, B. J.; Kunkel, D.; Linz, D. et al. (1997): "Violence in Television Programming Overall", *UCSB National Television Violence Study: Scientific Papers*, Newbury Park - California, Sage.

PART II

SERIAL KILLERS

Chapter 5

CONCEPT AND HISTORY OF THE SERIAL KILLER[*]

José Sanmartín
Queen Sofia Center for the Study of Violence &
Department of Philosophy of Science, University of Valencia, Spain

1. DEFINITION

Some murderers kill three or more victims, with a certain cooling-off period between them. These are the so-called "serial killers."
John Wayne Gacy, José Antonio Rodríguez Vega, and Christa Lehmann are three such cases.

2. JOHN WAYNE GACY

John Wayne Gacy was born in 1942 and did not exactly enjoy a happy childhood. His father was an alcoholic and used to beat him. He also received a heavy blow to the head in a playground accident involving a swing. As a result of this accident, he had frequent blackouts until it was discovered he had a blood clot on the brain, which was dissolved.

He married in 1964 and four years later was accused of having handcuffed and sodomized an employee. He was imprisoned in the psychiatric hospital of the State University of Iowa for 18 months.

After getting a divorce, John Wayne Gacy went to live in Chicago. In 1971 he again ran into trouble with the law after trying to force an adolescent to have sex with him, but the case was dismissed because the boy did not testify. Soon afterwards started the deadly chain of murders which led to Gacy's arrest in 1978.

During this period, Gacy started a construction business, working very hard and dedicating what little free time he had to humanitarian activities, organizing charity events, where he dressed up as Pogo the Clown, and donating the money raised to homeless children. He seemed a good man, deeply committed with other people's welfare. Reality, however, was

---

[*] Translated by Xavier De Jonge.

radically different, as he still found time for another type of activity. After building a crawl space under his home, he started to fill it with the bodies of young men that he had savagely murdered. Luring them to his house on the promise of money or a job, he handcuffed them, put a rope around their necks in which he had previously made two knots, inserted a stick in these knots and started turning it slowly. He often read Bible passages to his victims while he was strangling them in this way.

In all, John Wayne Gacy apparently killed 33 people. During his trial, his defense pleaded mental illness, alleging that he had multiple personalities as in the case of Dr. Jekyll and Mr. Hyde. The prosecutor, on the other hand, labeled him a psychopath. In the end, he was sentenced to death.

Gacy spent 14 years on death row, during which he painted, wrote, and also granted interviews to leading journalists, who turned him into a celebrity. In fact, he was the first serial killer to gain prominence in the media.

3. JOSE ANTONIO RODRIGUEZ VEGA

This Spaniard, who is still serving time, did not disguise himself as Pogo the Clown to do good deeds. He did not want to hide his face. In fact, his face was his greatest asset.

As a young man, Rodríguez Vega not only raped several women, but when he was arrested he succeeded in getting all but one to forgive him. His angelic face did not, however, keep him out of prison, for he served eight years.

After his release, he murdered at least 16 elderly women from April 1987 to April 1988. He consistently followed the same modus operandi. His good looks enabled him to gain the trust of these women, and as he was a bricklayer by profession, they usually asked him to carry out some construction work in their homes. He would then assault the women and strangle them slowly while raping them. He thus managed to murder at least 16 women, whose ages ranged from 61 to 93 years.

Rodríguez Vega was very organized in his crimes. First, he identified a potential victim and observed her until he knew her every habit. He then proceeded to establish contact, trying to gain the victim's trust with the aid of his appearance. When he gained entrance to the victim's home, he killed her. He did not go to great lengths to destroy evidence, although the age of his victims sometimes led to a clumsy diagnosis of death by natural causes. Finally, he was in the habit of collecting mementos from his victims. When he was arrested, police found a red room in his home in which he had arranged his souvenirs, from a television set to a plastic flower bouquet.

Rodríguez Vega was clearly sexually motivated. He did not kill to rob, all he took from the victims was some sort of trophy for himself. In the same way that some hunters have the heads of their prey mounted on walls, Rodríguez Vega decorated his red room with the souvenirs collected from his victims, which helped him to relive the excitement of the kill.

4. CHRISTA LEHMANN AND PARATHION

In Worms, Germany, on February 15, 1954, Annie Hamann died in the midst of violent convulsions after eating a chocolate she found in her refrigerator. The chocolate was a gift to her mother, Eva, from a neighbor called Christa Lehmann.

The circumstances of Annie's death were, to say the least, suspicious. All she had done was take a small bite from the chocolate, swallow part of it, and spit out the rest in disgust. Her dog had eaten the rejected chocolate and he, too, died shortly thereafter in convulsions.

Evidence of death by poisoning was overwhelming, but as had happened before, the chemical industry seriously challenged Toxicology.

For obvious reasons, the science of toxicology has always lagged behind the natural sciences. Once a new poison is discovered, toxicology sets out to develop procedures for detecting it in the body of a victim. Sometimes the pressure put on toxicology by the natural sciences is quite heavy. Thus, when toxicology had succeeded in finding ways of detecting arsenic and other mineral-metallic poisons, vegetal poisons such as nicotine started to appear. Later on, chemists and pharmacists again confounded toxicologists by developing synthetic poisons: barbiturates and tranquilizers. Regrettably, these historical changes always had one thing in common: invariably, some woman was ahead of her time and administered the newly discovered –and as yet impossible to detect– poison to her husband or some other person who aroused her anger. With the deaths of Annie Hamann and her dog, history again repeated itself.

That the unfortunate chocolate contained poison, was evident. What was not known at the time was what poison it contained, and how it had ended up in the chocolate. After due investigation, it was ruled out that the chocolate was poisoned by the company that produced it or the shop that sold it. Someone between the shop and Annie's refrigerator has introduced the poison in the chocolate. Attention turned to Christa Lehmann, and she finally confessed.

Christa Lehmann's life had been somewhat particular. She practically grew up without parents, marrying Karl Franz Lehmann, a bricklayer specialized in floors, in 1952. Together, they lived a golden age during the black market days after World War Two. However, they squandered the easy money in orgies, and when the lean years arrived, their relationship deteriorated into frequent and bitter rows, sometimes leading to physical violence. The sudden death of her husband, due to a stomach perforation apparently caused by his fondness for alcohol, returned Christa her freedom and she took full advantage of it, openly enjoying the company of other men. Only her father-in-law reprimanded her for her licentious behavior and, curiously, he too died suddenly while driving his bike, after having some yogurt for breakfast.

Christa then found a ready companion in Annie. Annie's mother Eva, however, considered Christa to be nothing less than the devil for Annie, dragging her into the depths of degradation. For that reason, Christa decided to take care of Eva, and gave her a chocolate. Eva, however, did not eat it and left it in the refrigerator.

All this information is known to us because Christa, in a remarkably cold display of remorselessness, volunteered it after being arrested. She also admitted to killing her husband and father-in-law.

She had used a new poison in the killings, a potent insecticide of widespread agricultural use and easy availability called E-605, or parathion.

Once more, a woman made history in toxicology, a science whose origins were closely linked with female murders. Suffice it to recall that it was Henry Fielding, the founder of the 18th century Bow Street Runners, who first called for scientific methods to be developed to verify the presence of poison in the body of a man who was thought to have been murdered by his wife. He declared that if the poison could be discovered and exposed, the woman would hang. However, a century would pass before there were, for the first time, reliable methods for detecting the poison of choice used by women for generations: arsenic.

5. IN SPITE OF EVERYTHING, THEY SAY THERE ARE NO FEMALE SERIAL KILLERS

I am sure that for many readers Christa Lehmann did not fit the conventional image of the serial killer. In fact, this image is so commonplace that the media often state that there are no female serial killers.

Now, this is not true, at least not as long as we define the serial killer, as we have done until now, as someone who kills three or more persons with a cooling-off period in between crimes. If we accept this definition, then the list of female serial killers is very long indeed.[1]

This is not to say that these women do not display a distinct criminal behavior. Their motive is usually money, which is not surprising given the traditional economic dependence of women on partners, husbands or not, who frequently maltreated them. For obvious reasons, they do not kill through brute force, nor do they use easily detectable instruments of death, such as knives or firearms. Rather, they use cunning and the stealth of poison. As the natural sciences discovered them, arsenic, nicotine and other vegetable poisons, synthetic pharmaceuticals, phytosanitary compounds, etcetera, all started to turn up in these women's crimes. These poisons are difficult to detect: toxicology initially often lacks proper detection techniques, and symptoms are often mistaken for those of diseases. Finally, once these women solve the problem that initially threatened them (usually, a brutal husband) they continue to kill, and for increasingly trivial reasons.[2]

There are several reasons why women are forgotten in the literature on serial killers. One may be that the history of mankind is so imbued with machismo that not only are women's positive contributions to civilization omitted, but also their *dark side*. The image of the serial killer as we know it now may also be the product of multiple interactions that have ended up excluding women from the ranks of these monsters.

6. 'CONSTRUCTING' THE SERIAL KILLER

In the eighties 23 movies on serial killers were produced. In the nineties, there were 54 movies. This does not include movies about mass killers[3] or, in general, horror movies about vampires, werewolves, zombies and the like.[4]

There is not one serial killer in recent North American history whose story has not been turned into a film.

The audiences from all over the world that have seen these movies, have seen a white male, aged between 30 and 40 years, and sexually deviant, who frequently kills his victims according to an elaborate ritual.

It is this interaction between the world of entertainment and communications, spectators, scientists, police and some serial killers themselves that has constructed a concept of the serial killer that is increasingly detailed: the previous and very generic definition of the serial killer has been enriched with more and more added notes. A serial killer is no longer someone who murders three or more victims with a cooling-off period between them, but someone who, in addition to the previous characteristics, is –at least– male, white, and sexually deviant.

However, the richer a definition becomes, the narrower is its field of application. For example, the new concept of the serial killer leaves out women. And if –exceptionally–women are included, it is because they commit serial murders with the same methods and for the same reasons as men do.[5]

7. TYPES OF SERIAL KILLERS

Using the new "constructed" concept of the serial killer, some researchers classify them in accordance with the place where they commit their crimes. Thus, there are serial killers that kill in very specific places, such as their own home or a hospital.[6] Some operate within the confines of a city or a region.[7] Others commit murders in different localities within one country[8], and finally others are true travelers, crossing various countries in search of victims.[9] To simplify, we might say there are *sedentary* serial killers, those that kill in a specific place, and *migrating* serial killers, that go from one place to another looking for victims.

Other researchers (Holmes & DeBurger, 1988) classify serial killers according to their motives. They thus distinguish between visionary, mission-oriented, power/control and hedonistic serial killers. The visionary serial killer follows orders, voices or visions related to the forces of good or evil.[10] The mission-oriented serial killer is one who believes he is ridding society of genuine human trash.[11] The power/control serial killer craves, above all, the satisfaction of dominating a helpless victim. Finally, the hedonistic serial killer is a sensation seeker, especially those sensations connected with sexual activity. Hedonistic killers with sexual motives are usually called "lust murderers."

Ressler[12] believes, as do the FBI, that all serial killers are motivated by deviant fantasies that are replayed in their imagination, often from as far back as their childhood (Ressler & Schachtman, 1992). These deviant fantasies contain strong sexual and violent components. There is, therefore, always an underlying sexual motive in their crimes –even when the murders are not accompanied by explicit sexual acts– because the killers are invariably driven by aberrant fantasies of a marked pornographic nature. Viewed this way, all serial killers (visionaries, power/control and mission-oriented) would be lust murderers.

Personally, I agree that deviant fantasies play an important role in serial killing (and in hyperviolent acts in general) but it should be remembered that in order to kill repeatedly and successively it is not sufficient to merely have fantasies. In our opinion, there must be some predispositions to murder.

8. PSYCHOTICS AND PSYCHOPATHS

Predispositions may take various forms, severe mental illness –such as a psychosis– being one of them. Or there may be a serious personality disorder, like psychopathy. It does certainly appear that if a serial killer is not a schizophrenic, he is a psychopath.

Still, this does not mean there are no social factors influencing the serial killer's behavior. There are, but always together with a psychosis or psychopathy. The predominant social factor is a childhood of rejection. Ed Kemper, who killed at least 10 people between 1964 and 1973, often decapitating them, is a textbook example of a serial killer who grew up feeling rejected by his family. Ed already was a giant at the age of 8, so much so that, according to his mother, he frightened his sisters and visitors. As a consequence, his mother kept him locked up in the basement for almost 8 months.

In short, we can classify serial killers according to their disorder. Each type of serial killer tends to kill in a very characteristic manner: the psychotics are very disorganized; the psychopaths, on the other hand, are very methodical. We can, therefore, separate serial killers into the *organized* and the *disorganized*, although there are occasionally *mixed* cases, i.e. partly organized and partly disorganized serial killers.

9. MODUS OPERANDI[13]

9.1. Before the murder

The psychotic serial killer tends to operate (like the visionary) under what he believes to be orders from superior entities such as God or Satan. He does not plan his crime beforehand, and does not pick his victims in a logical way. This is why he sometimes chooses a high-risk victim that puts up a fight, which forces the killer to inflict severe wounds and mutilations.

The psychopathic serial killer, on the contrary, plans his crimes with clearness of mind and attention to the smallest detail. He knows what he will do and does not want to fail. His longstanding deviant fantasies guide him in the selection of a victim. For instance, Ted Bundy, the prototypical organized serial killer, consistently chose girls with long, lank hair parted in the middle.[14] The organized serial killer not only chooses victims for a common physical feature, but he also chooses easily controllable victims. Absolute control over the victim is, moreover, one of the main objectives of the organized serial killer.

9.2. During the murder

As previously stated, both disorganized and organized serial killers commit crimes of a sexual nature. But also here do we see marked differences between the two types. The organized serial killer generally rapes his victim before killing her. The disorganized killer, however, tends to have sex with dead or completely inanimate victims. "El Arropiero," who I described in footnote 8, came across an elderly woman of 68 years in the night of 23 November 1969. He asked her if she wanted to have sex with him. She indignantly refused, whereupon he beat her to death with a brick and threw her dead body into a dry streambed. Seeing that the body was visible from above, he descended into the streambed and before hiding the body from view, raped it. During the following nights he returned to the site to again rape the poor woman's corpse until it was found by children.

As the organized serial killer, contrary to the disorganized one, wants to control his victims, it is not surprising that he keeps them alive long enough to act out the different aspects that make up his aberrant fantasies.

Carrying out these fantasies usually also requires the use of instruments or tools. Not surprisingly, the organized serial killer, who follows a previously thought-out plan and wants to control his victims, carries a sort of kit, containing materials such as rope, handcuffs, scalpels, etcetera. To the contrary, the disorganized killer uses anything that comes to hand. If he finds a knife in the victim's home, he may stick it in her chest and leave it there. That is precisely where another important difference lies. The disorganized serial killer will not bother to wipe fingerprints, hide the body or take other steps to hinder the investigation. But the organized serial killer will make life as hard as possible for the police, so much so that occasionally his confession adds new murders to those he is originally accused of.

9.3. After the murder

Organized and disorganized serial killers show differences in behavior after committing a murder. The organized serial killer will take home a souvenir from the victim, such as underwear, necklaces or shoes, etcetera. Some even keep body parts. They are their private trophies, and they will not hesitate to adorn their favorite room with them, as José A. Rodríguez Vega did.

Subsequently, in a move that is his potential downfall, the organized serial killer may follow the progress of the investigation, not because he is afraid of being arrested, but because he enjoys continuing to control the situation. In this regard, Ressler[15] recounts the horrible case of a hospital ambulance driver who would kidnap his victims from the parking lot of a restaurant and take them to another place to rape and kill them. He would then leave the bodies partially exposed and call the police to report them. This is not the behavior of an organized serial killer, but of a man with an overriding need to control. What he really loved doing was drive quickly back to the hospital after a murder and then, when police discovered the body and called for an ambulance, rush out to the scene and take his own victim back to the hospital!

10. EVIL

Disorganized serial killers do not frighten us as much as psychopathic serial killers, perhaps because the disorganized killers are in the grip of serious mental disorders. They are beyond the thin red line that separates them –the "crazies"– from us –the sane. We are put at ease by knowing the principal motive that forces them to act as they do, and our own mental health seems to guarantee that we will never commit such aberrant acts ourselves.

But the organized serial killers are deeply unsettling to us. Like us, they do not suffer from any serious mental disorder that prevents them from knowing what they do. What makes them different from us is that they feel no regret for what they do.

Indeed, organized serial killers are very coldhearted throughout the different stages of their crimes, and they do not seem to empathize with their victims at any time. They treat them as predators would their prey. It is as if their victims do not belong to the same species. They play with them like a cat plays with a mouse. They want to keep them alive as long as possible in order to prolong the pleasure of total control and domination. They kill when they want to kill, when they believe they have reached the summit of pleasure, which almost always coincides with the union of sex and death.

11. WHAT MAKES THEM BEHAVE LIKE THAT?

Most researchers try to explain the behavior of organized serial killers through a series of social factors. Foremost among these factors is growing up in a dysfunctional home, with –at least– emotional abuse. Hickey[16] attaches great importance to the fact that these murderers overwhelmingly suffered rejection and as a result grew up deeply frustrated. Ressler[17] shares the same opinion.

Personally, I am not convinced. In another book[18], I wrote that aberrant behavior such as kidnapping, sodomy, murder, butchering, and keeping adolescents' heads in the fridge in order to have oral sex with them, is difficult to comprehend as the result of frustration caused by rejection by the mother.

These individuals meet the criteria of Hare's Psychopathy Checklist-revised almost to the letter. For this reason, we have divided serial killers in groups based on the type of disorder they suffer. And psychopathy is not a mental disorder, but a personality disorder, whose symptoms may be caused by cerebral dysfunctions.

In this book, Adrian Raine tells how the orbitofrontal cortex of impulsive murderers shows low levels of activity. Obviously, an organized serial killer is not impulsive. He plans his crimes, and thus uses this region of the brain as much as, or even more than, any normal person. Raine's brain scans of murderers of this type prove this point.

I would venture to suggest that the anomaly we are looking for is not in the orbitofrontal but in the ventromedial cortex. It is currently coming to light that within the frontal lobes, the prefrontal dorsolateral cortex is the center charged with making plans that the orbitofrontal cortex then decides to carry out or not. The ventromedial cortex, for its part, assigns emotional meaning to our perceptions and actions. A dysfunctional ventromedial cortex would, then, cause emotions not to be assigned to actions, or to be assigned incorrectly. This might explain the psychopath's coldness and, ultimately, lack of empathy (See Sanmartín, 2000b).

I advance the hypothesis that certain social factors that have a low threshold, i.e. social factors that would have little or no influence in a normal person's behavior, have a great impact in organized serial killers.

12. A THEORY OF THE BEHAVIOR OF ORGANIZED SERIAL KILLERS[19]

I will try to bring together all that has been said before into an explanatory model of the behavior of the organized serial killer.

Obviously, I believe it is very important that there be a predisposition toward violent behavior. This predisposition would be a serious personality disorder, namely psychopathy.

Some social factors usually influence these individuals during their childhoods and adolescence. In particular, they suffer emotional abuse. They feel undervalued or rejected. And they start to escape into fantasies that allow them to overcome, at least in their imagination, their specific frustrations.

We all have fantasies. But the fantasies that these individuals begin to recreate in their imagination, especially from adolescence onwards, tend to have very strong sexually deviant components, combined with heavy doses of violence. Moreover, as adolescents these individuals condition themselves by masturbating while fantasizing. Thus, the fantasies become associated with pleasure.

The organized serial killer recreates his particular fantasies using the materials provided by the sources that feed his imagination. These sources include pornographic magazines and comic books, books on the occult, and –dare we say– the images from the movies, television, computers and game pads.

In no way am I claiming that reading or viewing these materials will turn a normal person into a predator who preys on his own species. What I do believe they do is mold the deviant fantasies, into which the psychopaths retreat from their frustrations. So it should come as no surprise, given the globalization of the audiovisual media, that the deviant fantasies of psychopaths from different and distant countries are quite similar.

Until recently the organized serial killer was considered to be something American or, at most, British. We now know there have been such murderers in the United States, Mexico, Columbia, Brazil, Spain, the United Kingdom, Germany, Russia, Pakistan, etcetera. Why? Perhaps these serial killers have similar *modi operandi* because they have tapped the same sources to feed their deviant fantasies. The screen has fed them.

In short, I am defending a model in which a predisposition (psychopathy), accompanied by certain social factors (mainly emotional rejection), leads to certain frustrations which the individual tries to overcome by retreating into deviant fantasies.

Finally, what may cause a psychopath to act out his fantasies? I do not think there is a universal answer. The reason may be different in each individual. Like the good psychopaths they are, they all believe themselves superior. As they believe themselves superior, everything is frustrating to them, they feel abused by everything and everyone because they cannot reach the goals they think they are ideally suited to. They are angry at the world. It is only normal that they harbor feelings of revenge as a result of this anger. Anything, then, may light the fuse of their revenge and make them unload all the violence which they experienced and –until that moment– only used to the fullest in their deviant inner fantasies.

NOTES

1 On the use of poison, I recommend chapter 3 of Thorwald, J. (1964).

2 In 1949, Frenchwoman Marie Besnard was accused of killing 13 people, using arsenic. She is thought to have poisoned her second husband driven by an irrepressible passion toward a German employee. The other suspected victims were poisoned either because they hindered her romance with the German or for financial reasons. The lack of information regarding arsenic's behavior and her defense lawyers' competence allowed her to walk free in 1961, after three trials. She was known as the "Black Widow," after the much feared spider that kills its victims with poison.

The same sobriquet has been applied recently to Margarita Sánchez Gutiérrez, author of some eight poison killings during the Olympic Games in Barcelona.

Margarita Sánchez, also nicknamed "squint" because of the extreme strabismus that affected her right eye, was raised in an environment rife with financial hardship and physical abuse. Her subsequent relationship with her husband, a subway driver, took on a noted aversive character, which became worse shortly before he died of a strange illness, the same illness in fact which killed three more (two neighbors and a brother-in-law) and which three others escaped *in extremis*. Except in her husband's case, the "Black Widow" always benefited economically from the deaths, although the final amount did not exceed $12,000. The poison she used was a type of medicine that, when taken in high doses, has a devastating effect on the circulatory system.

3 A mass killer is not a serial killer. Whereas the serial killer kills his victims one after the other, spacing the murders, a mass killer kills several people at once or in a short period of time. Mass killers are predominantly white males, use firearms, have feelings of failure that cause them to seek revenge, are mentally ill and end their killing sprees by committing suicide.

4 See Hickey (1997), p. 4.

5 Between 1989 and 1990, Aileen Carol Wuornos killed at least 7 men. There have been many women who killed more people. What makes Aileen C. Wuornos' case interesting is that her motives for killing and her methods were very similar to those of the usual serial killer.

Aileen was born in Michigan in 1956. Her parents were very young: her mother was 16, her father 19. The marriage lasted but a few months. Her father was jailed for robbery and rape, and committed suicide in prison. Her mother abandoned her when she was 6 months old. From then onwards, she was raised by her grandparents.

According to Aileen, she was raped at age 13 and got pregnant. After giving her child up for adoption, she started to live anywhere and nowhere, and began taking marihuana, acid and mescaline. Later she worked as a prostitute and was repeatedly abused and raped. At age 22 she had already made 6 suicide attempts.

When she was 25, she was jailed in connection with a robbery. While in prison (14 months) she received various punishments for improper conduct. After being released she began having lesbian sex and also started her career as a serial killer.

Aileen killed 7 men between 1989 and 1990. She behaved like a male serial killer: she carefully selected strangers (driving an expensive car was one of her selection criteria), and was dominant and violent with her victims. She tried not to leave fingerprints, and her crimes were motivated by deviant sexual tendencies.

6 Consider the chilling case of Edson Izidoro Gimaraes, the Brazilian nurse who was arrested in 1999 and confessed having killed 6 patients, although the true number of victims is probably close to 150.

7 Andrei Romanovich Chikatilo, the "Monster of Rostov", was arrested in 1990 and accused of 36 murders, to which he voluntarily added another 18. Most of his victims were women, whose uteri he tore out in true Jack the Ripper fashion, and boys and girls, whose genitals he destroyed with his teeth.

He committed all his murders in Rostov and the surrounding region. His arrest in the midst of *perestroika* was eagerly depicted by the former communists as proof of the innate degeneracy of the capitalist democracy that was taking root in Russia at the time. It should not be forgotten that true socialism does not recognize mental illness, but rather social illness, and that communism, by its very essence, was the proper recipe for avoiding the kind of serious social deviations that might give rise to a monster like Chikatilo.

However, Chikatilo had been imitating Jack the Ripper since 1978. He was, therefore, not a product of the recent changes, but a clear example of the fact that this type of murderers can occur anywhere and in any political system. In fact, it was socialist dogmatism that prevented him being arrested earlier, being as he was a humble functionary and Communist Party member.

8 Manuel Delgado Villegas, nicknamed "el Arropiero" because he was the son of an *arrope* vendor [note: *arrope* is a typically Spanish dark sweet syrup made from grapes and honey and which may also contain pumpkin and melon peel] was a schizophrenic who committed at least 22 murders between 1964 and 1971. Once he was detained, the police took him to various Spanish locations where he claimed to have killed someone.

9 Luis Alfredo Garavito's may be such a case. Garavito was detained in October 1999 and has confessed killing about 140 children and adolescents since 1992. Most bodies were found close to some 60 cities in at least 11 of Columbia's 32 provinces, but it is thought he may also have killed in Ecuador.

Luis Alfredo Garavito is the eldest of seven children. As a young boy he was repeatedly beaten by his father and also raped by two neighbors. As an adolescent he started consuming great amounts of alcohol. He underwent psychiatric treatment for depression and several suicide attempts.

Garavito's victims were mainly boys between 8 and 16 years old, the sons of street vendors or homeless people. Garavito pretended to be a beggar, a street vendor, or sometimes even a lecturer speaking in schools on behalf of foundations dedicated to child protection or the care of elderly people. He lured his victims with sweets, money, or alcohol. Alcohol also appears to have been present in many of his crimes, as Garavito himself said he was completely drunk in most of his murders.

10 Spain has recently known a case of a visionary serial murderer who, according to his own statements, killed 15 people. With one exception, all his victims were beggars, indigents or socially marginal people. The killer in question is Francisco García Escalero, a schizophrenic who mixed Rohipnol with wine. Following the dictates of voices that demanded more blood, Escalero –aka "*El matamendigos*" or "the Killer of Beggars"– went as far as to dig up corpses from a cemetery in Madrid and to lie down with them. As it happens, this cemetery was a constant factor in his life: he lived very close to it during

his childhood and adolescence, and he liked to stroll alone among the tombs, preferably at night.

11 According to Egger (1998), chapter 4, serial killers usually choose as victims the "less dead." This term denotes that those victims are frequently people that are very vulnerable by virtue of their profession, age or situation, such as prostitutes, homosexuals or indigents, whose death may carry less social weight than that of a "normal" person.

12 Robert K. Ressler, FBI expert for 20 years, was instrumental in the creation of the FBI's Behavioral Sciences Unit, and was an outstanding criminal profiler of serial killers, contributing to the arrest of many from their ranks.

13 See chapter 6 of Ressler & Schachtman (1992).

14 Ted Bundy is thought to have kidnapped, tortured, raped, killed and partially devoured some 40 women between 1974 and 1978. However, he did not have the appearance of a monster. On the contrary, thanks to his good looks, elegance, and verbal skills, the media turned him into a real "dandy" of crime, "a Mr. Nice Guy, almost a benign killer, a good lover who would kill his victims quickly" (Ressler & Schachtman, 1992, p. 72).
Bundy, however, was a true monster who meticulously planned his lethal actions: he would choose a victim, approach her with a false cast on one arm in which he also hid a short crowbar, ask her to open the door of his car, and when she bowed to do so, he would push her into the car and kidnap her. He would then perform all types of sadist sexual practices on her, including sodomy, kill her, mutilate her sexual organs and bite off pieces of flesh from her belly and thighs. When committing these atrocities, Bundy said, he felt like a vampire following orders from superior entities.
Bundy was cold and devoid of empathy. He did not show any kind of remorse after his arrest. In addition, Bundy was a master manipulator who systematically and methodically tried to cheat on everybody. In short, he was a typical psychopath.

15 Ressler & Schachtman (1992), pp. 136-137.

16 Hickey (1997), p. 87: "For serial murderers the most common effect of childhood traumatization manifested is rejection, including rejection by relatives and parent(s). It must be emphasized that an unstable, abusive home has been reported as one of the major forms of rejection."

17 Ressler, R. K. & Schachtman, T. (1992): *Whoever Fights Monsters*, New York, St. Martin's Paperbacks, pp. 83-84: "Nonetheless, though the homes [of the serial killers Ressler interviewed] seemed to outward appearances to be normal, they were in fact dysfunctional. ... Half had parents who had been involved in criminal activities. Nearly 70 percent had a familial history of alcohol or drug abuse. All the murderers –every single one– were subjected to serious *emotional* [his emphasis] abuse during their childhoods. And all of them developed into what psychiatrists label as sexually dysfunctional adults, unable to sustain a mature, consensual relationship with another adult. ... Relationships between our subjects and their mothers were uniformly cool, distant, unloving, neglectful. ... These children grew up in an environment in which their own actions were ignored, and in which there were no limits set on their behavior."

18 Sanmartín (2000a), chapter 2.

19 Hickey (1997), chapter 4 , presents an extensive overview of the different theories about serial killers. I can accept the Trauma-Control Model, up to a certain point. I disagree with the marked environmentalist nature that Hickey ascribes to this behavior: he believes that only social factors can lead to frustration and low self-esteem which, with the help of deviant fantasies, lead to murder, and more murder. Nor am I convinced that these murderers have low self-esteem. Rather, I believe they if they feel frustrated by everything and everyone, it is precisely because they feel superior, not because they feel inferior.

REFERENCES

Cleckley, H. (1976): *The mask of sanity* (5th ed.), St. Louis, MO, Mosby.

Cooke, D. J.; Forth, A. E. & Hare, R. D. (eds.) (1998): *Psychopathy: Theory, research, and implications for society*, Dordrecht, The Netherlands, Kluwer.

Egger, S. A. (1990): *Serial Murder: An Elusive Phenomenon*, Westport, CT, Praeger.

Egger, S. A. (1998): *The Killers Among Us*, London, Prentice Hall.

Giannangelo, S. J. (1996): *The Psychopathology of Serial Murder: A theory of violence*, Westport, CT, Praeger.

Hare, R. D. (1993): *Without Conscience: The disturbing world of the psychopaths among us*, New York, Pocket Books, reissued in 1998 by Guilford Press.

Hickey, E. W. (1997): *Serial Murderers and their Victims*, Belmont, CA., Wadsworth Publ. Co.

Holmes, R. M. & DeBurger, J. (1988): *Serial Murder*, NewBury Park, CA., Sage.

Pérez Abellán, Francisco (1998): *Crónica de la España negra*, Madrid, Espasa-Calpe.

Pérez Abellán, Francisco (1999): *¿Quién lo hizo?*, Madrid, Espasa-Calpe.

Pérez Abellán, Francisco (2000): *Ellas matan mejor*, Madrid, Espasa-Calpe.

Ressler, R. K. & Schachtman, T. (1992): *Whoever Fights Monsters*, New York, St. Martin's Paperbacks.

Sanmartín, J. (2000a): *La violencia y sus claves*, Barcelona, Ariel.

Sanmartín, J. (2000b): "Las raíces de la violencia", *Debats*, 70/71, pp. 8-25.

Skrapec, C. (1994): "The female serial killer: An evolving criminality", in H. Birch (ed.), *Moving Targets. Women, Murder and Representation*, Berkeley, Los Angeles, University of California Press.

Skrapec, C. (1996): "The Sexual Component of Serial Murder", in T. O'Reilly-Fleming, *Serial and Mass Murder: Theory, Research and Policy*, Toronto, Canadian Scholars' Press.

Thorwald, J. (1964): *Das Jahrhundert der Detektive*, Zürich, Drömer.

Chapter 6

MOTIVES OF THE SERIAL KILLER

Candice A. Skrapec
Department of Criminology, California State University Fresno, Fresno, California, USA

The mind is its own place, and in it self
Can make a Heav'n of Hell, a Hell of Heav'n.

Here we may reign secure, and in my choice
To reign is worth ambition though in hell:
Better to reign in hell, than serve in heav'n.

Milton, *Paradise Lost*, bk. I, l.247

1. IS EVIL A CHOICE?

For many people, social scientists and laymen alike, serial murderers have been summarily relegated to the realm of evil. The very existence of serial killers[1] turns up the rhetoric on evil. Why would someone be motivated to kill repeatedly if not as a manifestation of some evil force? However, just as we observe the behaviors of most serial killers to be "crazy" –yet not most killers themselves– we find ourselves in a similar position with respect to the evil of their deeds. While we may describe the series of killings as evil, the perpetrators are of decidedly human substance. Their "evil" is borne of their willful intent to destroy human life. Serial murderers do not inhabit a kind of "otherness," but rather reveal extreme aspects of our very selves. My own experiences with them have taught me to accept them –but not what they do– unconditionally, as human beings. This permits a window into their killings; and access to a comprehensibility with regard to their motives.

Any arrogance that the title of this article might suggest attaches to a confidence in our tenacious scientific curiosity, not to our current level of understanding of why serial murderers do what they do. This is a paper which, at the outset, acknowledges it is about a subject that we are never likely to completely understand: why some people kill repeatedly—not in

Violence and Psychopathy, edited by Raine & Sanmartin,
Kluwer Academic/Plenum Publishers, New York, 2001.

the service of a political ideology, nor as a function of murder-as-occupation, but rather for perverse personal gratification. Indeed, why should serial murder be any more comprehensible than any other human behavior, which is, after all, a veritable black box of complexity? This disclaimer notwithstanding, we have learned much about behavior from a multitude of disciplines, all of which bears upon our understanding of serial murder.

2. INTRODUCTION

The rarity of serial murder is not an argument for directing our research into other areas of violence. Just as extreme points on a continuum help to define the center, knowledge about serial murder—as an extreme form of violent behavior—better informs our understanding of the human condition. With each incident of violence that comes to our attention we hear ourselves reacting with the same question: Why? And our thinking inevitably takes us to the realization that the answer requires an understanding of the motive forces that underlie the violent behavior. Motive is the heart of the enigma of violence; and so with serial murder, one of its most extreme forms.

By and large, serial murderers have not changed much over time. We are in witness today of the same kinds of atrocities visited upon victims in earlier centuries. Apart from adopting the nuances of their respective times (e.g., in the 1990s, making videotaped recordings of their murders) the crimes of serial killers have remained remarkably similar over hundreds of years. We see much the same kinds of behavior by serial killers over time, from which may be inferred persisting motivational dynamics.

What motive forces underlie a series of murders? The *Oxford English Dictionary* speaks of motive as an inward prompting or impulse that influences volition. The question of motivation—what causes a person to behave in a particular way—is answered in terms of antecedent conditions that activate and direct specific behavior. (Reeve, 1992) Early accounts of serial murders described them as random and motiveless killings. The headlines of newspaper articles and television news stories about newly apprehended serial killers regularly included the term "senseless." An American television documentary on serial killers was even titled "Murder: No Apparent Motive."[2] Most of these murders are, however, neither random nor lacking in discernible motive. Our experience with serial killers has shown that they tend to selectively target their victims and do so in the service of some inextinguishable personal need.

3. THE MULTIDIMENSIONALITY OF MOTIVE

It is not enough to ask what energizes the serial murderer's efforts to kill; we must understand why he[3] kills in the first place, and then why he continues to do so. A growing literature on behavior teaches that biological factors predispose certain individuals to act in violent ways. How impulsive we tend to be is, in part, a function of levels of serotonin in the brain (which alcohol consumption can lower); how aggressive, a function of levels of circulating testosterone (which can be raised with steroids). Years of research situate the roots of episodic violence in neurobiology; the result of brain dysfunction.

Paleopsychology offers another order of explanation of aggressive behavior where the power of socialization is effectively nulled by a regression to more primitive levels of functioning. Bailey (1987) sees the stalk-attack-kill fixed action patterns of predatory animals –albeit in fragmented form– in chronically violent humans; people behaving in phylogenetically regressed ways. These individuals operate according to compelling and inborn motivational forces. In their discussion of violent offenders, Wrangham and Peterson (1996) make reference to evolutionary roots of "demonic" males (and females), individuals whose primitive temperamental traits lend themselves to vicious, lethal aggression, and whose more highly developed human ingenuity make them especially dangerous. Bailey posits that the Ted Bundys of the world are not distinctive for their proclivities (which are a function of a primitive survival blueprint built into neurological structures and pathways), but rather they are remarkable for releasing those innate tendencies – for lacking normal inhibitions. In committing their crimes, they are discharging normal selfish, primitive drives. They are, in a sense, "victims" of their urges, by virtue of neurological dysfunction.

Some of the propositions of paleopsychology are supported by findings of biological research on violent offenders. Measures of psychophysiological arousal among these individuals tend to reveal distinctive baseline activity consistent with underarousal – reduced skin conductance rates, heart rates, and cortical activity patterns. Raine (1994) reports PET scan differences between single-incident and serial murderers in the activity levels of the prefrontal cortex. Typically, single murderers –like the attention-deficit disordered child– show depressed levels of arousal in this region of the brain that is responsible for executive functions like planning and regulating behavior. Multiple murderers, on the other hand, show a substantial degree of prefrontal activity (even though other psychophysiological indicators are depressed). These observations are consistent with our experience with the two types of killers in that single murderers tend to kill on impulse while the multiple murderer usually kills after much deliberation and planning. Our thinking about the motivations that underlie serial murder must take into account the psychophysiological parameters that prime some individuals to act in violent ways.

Raine (1993) offers a persuasive case for conceptualizing criminality as a clinical disorder. As a syndrome, he describes criminality as the product of specific biological (including genetic) predispositions toward, for example, impulsive and aggressive actions, and their interactions with psychological and social factors. Physiological processes form the substance and shape the contours of the biological substrate upon which an environment acts. Hence, the kind of "poker hand" of criminality described by Sarnoff Mednick.[4] In order to become criminal, one must have all of the requisite cards for the "flush." These might include low levels of serotonin, abnormally high levels of testosterone, and a formative environment that activates and directs criminal behaviors. An integrated (read interactive) model is capable of explaining the complexity of serial murder; single-factor or single-paradigm theories are not, nor are multivariable analyses that combine elements in an additive manner. The entity as a whole –the serial killer– is greater than the sum of its parts. Thus, the motive forces that propel his actions are multidimensional.

While it appears that most serial killers are predatory criminals, some kill as a function of opportunity, responding to situations in which they find themselves. The opportunist lacks the kind of preconceived cognitive map that guides the predator to his prey. He reacts to a particular situation by killing. His murders are not planned but rather the product of momentary impulse. While the predatory offender may also kill without premeditation in response to "a moment," he invests much of himself planning his crimes and actively seeking out those he can violate in the service of some rational or irrational need. With single-minded determination he creates his opportunities to kill.

In general, the purpose of behavior is to fulfill our desires or satisfy our needs. Individual serial killers, accordingly, do what works for them. Violence has utility. Modus operandi, the method or means by which a series of murders is accomplished, can provide critical clues about underlying motive. What an offender does –and does not do– in the commission of his crimes reveals much information about him, including the emotional underpinnings of the acts of murder. Fear, rage, disdain, sadism, and the like can be inferred from behavioral evidence at the crime scene. Subjecting victims to a degree of violence that far exceeds what is necessary to kill – that is, to "overkill"– constitutes enraged punctuation of, perhaps, a need to punish the victim (or what the victim represents to the perpetrator).

While the brutal and repetitive aspects of the killings suggest psychological disturbance in the offenders, the most seriously disturbed behaviors are most often *not* the product of the most serious kinds of psychopathology – at least not according to the conventional standards by which we currently conceptualize and define mental disorders (e.g., the Diagnostic and Statistical Manual of Mental Disorders-IV) (Dietz, 1986). Relatively few known serial killers have been clinically diagnosed as psychotic. Indeed, it is the absence of major mental illness –the fact that they are in touch with reality– that enables most serial murderers to commit their series of murders before or without being detected. Yet certainly, the serial killer is mentally disordered. If not psychosis, then what is the nature of the psychopathology from which most serial killings emerge?

A review of the literature on serial killers indicates that they run the gamut of what is psychopathologically possible. However, consistent with reports of other researchers and clinicians, the author's familiarity with a number of serial murderers and their case histories suggests that psychopathy –a "less serious" mental disorder– or at least psychopathic features, have a major role in the psychological makeup of these offenders. Primary psychological and behavioral criteria for psychopathy (e.g., lack of emotional empathy; lack of remorse; longstanding pattern of antisocial behavior) are evidenced in the majority of serial killers. The failure to be effectively socialized –not unrelated to the offender's lack of emotional empathy and inability to experience remorse– goes far to enable the serial killer to carry out his series of murders. Although we must remain mindful that not all serial killers are psychopaths and certainly only few psychopaths are serial killers, our studies of serial murderers reveal psychopathy rather than psychosis as the dominant psychopathology. Decades of research by Hare (e.g., 1993; 1970) support a neurobiological basis for the emotional deficits of the psychopath as they relate to his apparent inability to experience emotional empathy or to feel guilt for his antisocial acts.

On the other hand, it may be that psychiatry is not currently equipped to adequately conceptualize, and therefore, categorize the behaviors of individuals who make a criminal career out of murdering people for personal gratification. Clinical diagnoses are insufficient to explain the apparent need of a person to kill repeatedly. We need instead to better acquaint ourselves with the individual serial murderer: to examine the world as he experiences it. Anguished memories, distorted beliefs, and unresolved conflicts serve to organize the experiences of his life. On both a conscious and unconscious level, they direct his murderous behavior – and it is his behavior that provides us with a partial view through to his motivation.

Motivation is a multidimensional construct. This paper takes the position that serial murderers are individuals who are biologically predisposed to antisocial behavior; biologically primed for violence. Their psychological makeup, including their psychopathology, shapes how they perceive, organize, and evaluate the experiences of their lives. Most specifically, their proclivities to violence are activated and/or enhanced by the subjective experiences of their lives.

Motive implies cognitively directed action, at both conscious and unconscious levels of brain function. Studies on the biology of violence elucidate the mechanisms by which certain individuals are predisposed to and engage in violent behavior; this paper examines the cognitive outcome of such predisposition: how serial killers experience their world; and specifically, what the repeated acts of killing mean to the killers themselves.

4. MOTIVATIONAL IMPERATIVES

Rarely do we see serial murderers cease killing of their own accord. Heriberto Seda (the *Zodiac Killer* in New York City in 1990) and Edmund Emil Kemper III (the *Co-Ed Killer* in California in the 1970s) are exceptions(–which, as such, make them important to our understanding of serial murder). A much more common scenario, however, is that the killing career ends as the result of successful intervention by law enforcement. Most serial killers do not stop until they are stopped. This would appear to speak to the compelling and intractable nature of the killings for the perpetrator. Unlike serial rapists who may kill one or more victims because the violence of the crime escalates to a point resulting in death, or who may kill victims in order to reduce the chances of their apprehension, serial killers appear to need the corpse, implying an imperative to kill.

The murders of some serial murderers are rational, instrumental crimes such as schemes of serial murder as means to profit. The "black widow" phenomenon, in which (usually) a woman murders a number of spouses or suitors is perhaps the best known example of serial murder for financial gain. We are, however, much more familiar with series of murders with an emotive current and in which victims are sexually violated in various ways. And even then, the killings may only be incidental to the offender's motive. The 1929 killings by Düsseldorf's Peter Kürten appear to have been motivated by sexual gratification. Although his assaults resulted in the death of many of his victims, this was not his intent. Kürten became sexually aroused by the flow of blood that resulted from striking his victims with various implements. The number of blows was determined by how much time it took for him to reach orgasm. The greater the number of delivered blows, the greater was the likelihood the assault resulted in death. The murders were thus not by design, but rather the by-product of a paraphilia. We do not know how many serial murderers operate in this kind of mode, but the fact of their existence imposes a caveat upon our assessments of motive. To add another dimension of complexity, there are offenders whose killings could be also categorized as paraphilic, but for whom it is the act of killing itself that is eroticized (Money, 1990).

Serial murder includes, but is in no way limited to, sexual homicides. Even in cases where sexual violation is apparent, we cannot assume that the primary motive force is sexual gratification. In her discussion of motive in serial killings that involve sexual violation of victims, Skrapec (1996) distinguishes serial sexual homicide and sexualized serial homicide. Serial sexual murder implies sexual motive. The offender is killing for an orgasm, which he may experience before, during, and/or after the death of the victim. This is different from sexualized serial murder where although the modus operandi includes sexual violation of victims, the murders are driven by a desire or need to kill; that he does so in a manner that is sexually gratifying is secondary. This is not to say, in either case, that the driving motive is sexual. It is to say that we need to examine the role played by sexually assaultive behaviors in both types of offenses.

Historically, gender differences among serial killers have manifested themselves through such aspects as physical strength, with males generally better able and more inclined to use physical force as well as more visceral means (e.g., strangulation rather than suffocation). In her examination of female serial killers, Skrapec (1994) argues that while male and female offenders generally kill in different ways (although there are signs this may be changing, with females beginning to adopt more male-like means), the motives for killing are essentially the same. In both cases, the series of murders are perpetrated in the service of self-preservation: they are offensive acts driven by defensive imperatives. For both genders, killing is life-sustaining.

It is a strong contention of this paper that we cannot claim any understanding of the motives of serial killers without immersing ourselves into their subjective experiences. Learning about the details of their lives, including their killings –and how they experience them– locates for us a point of access to their motivation to kill and kill again.

5. THE SCHOLARLY INVESTIGATION OF MOTIVE

In investigating crimes, police are concerned with the motives of perpetrators; understanding why a crime was committed can implicate specific suspects as well as rule out unlikely individuals. In the scholarly investigation of the phenomenon of serial murder, motivation of offenders has, similarly, been the focus of much attention. Typologies of serial murderers have been constructed based upon categories of assumed motives of offenders. One of the main problems with such typologies is the recurring fact of overlap between established categories. A particular serial murderer might well fit several categories. How are we to know by his criminal behaviors that his crimes are primarily driven by a need to kill or for sexual gratification? Are the crimes those of a serial sexual murderer or a sexual serial murderer? Another and more troubling problem is the matter of determining motive in the first place. How are we in a position to assess motive without understanding what the series of murders actually accomplishes (or, does not accomplish!) for the perpetrator?

The task of elucidating the motive forces underlying serial murder in such a manner that evinces its meaning cannot rely upon traditional clinical and psychometric approaches. An alternative approach is called for; one that uncovers how serial murderers experience repeated acts of murder. The author was inspired to apply the phenomenological method as the result of statements made by serial killer Edmund Emil Kemper III. California's 1970s "Co-Ed Killer" challenged a veteran crime-reporter –to whom he had given an exclusive interview after his conviction on eight murder counts– for not asking the kinds of questions he had expected: "What is it like to have sex with a dead body?" By not asking such questions we preserve illusions that serial killers bear no likeness to us. Ed Kemper, however, has given us a way to "find" him amongst ourselves.

The methodology used in the study –empirical phenomenology– focused on an individual's experiences in order to gather comprehensive descriptions that provided the basis for a structural analysis representing the essence of his experiences. Put another way, the underlying structures of an experience were determined by interpreting an individual's narrative about the situations in which the experience occurred. Personal narratives reveal the meanings that organize an individual's life –whether they are derived from actual lived-experiences or whether the individual fabricates experiences and incorporates them into his narrative– ostensibly *because* they are meaningful to him.

Is there an inner narrative which drives the serial murderer to kill and kill again? The aim of the study was to determine what the experience of repeatedly killing means to individuals who have had that experience. The task required examining each act of murder in terms of what it meant to the murderer, being mindful to identify common themes across the series of murders. Documented elsewhere, Skrapec (1997) details the intensive semi-structured interviews with five incarcerated serial murderers. What follows are highlights from these interviews that most specifically bear upon the motives to kill.

6. DOMINANT THEMES AND EMOTIONAL MEANINGS

In detailing their crimes, all subjects spoke matter-of-factly about unspeakable things. They were not at all apprehensive about revealing the most reprehensible aspects of their criminal exploits. As the five subjects talked about their killings there emerged three dominant themes reflecting powerful intrapsychic forces; impelling their acts of murder. Threads of these themes permeated virtually all matters they discussed. The three themes are not, on the surface at least, such as would distinguish these serial murderers from other people. What is striking, however, is the degree to which or the manner in which subjects related to these dimensions. In recounting their killings, each subject revealed extreme if not oblique leanings in the areas of entitlement, empowerment, and vitality. The dynamics of these themes appeared to organize their killing experiences, and indeed, the lived meanings of their lives.

6.1. Entitlement

As they recalled their murders, the predominant theme across all subjects was that of entitlement. In general, each subject appeared to maintain a distorted place for himself vis-à-vis the rest of the world in that whatever he did was essentially justified by virtue of the fact that it was he who did it. Even when a subject recalled a situation and would himself remark upon how despicable his actions were, his vocal tone if not his actual words to a frequently startling degree revealed a sense of righteous indignation on his part. While he could acknowledge his wrongdoing on a cognitive level –in that he knows that there are social and legal rules proscribing what he did– underlying this awareness appeared to be a personal conviction that his actions were justified. There was a disjunction between the cognitive awareness he has of the wrongfulness of his conduct and the emotional meaning he attached to his behavior. This is the individual who loses patience with those of us who cannot understand that even though he is "technically" the perpetrator of the harmful deed. He is really the victim doling out due punishment.

All five subjects experienced themselves, first and foremost, as victims. The objective reality of their experiences is irrelevant. That they experienced themselves as victims was their reality. That they victimized others was not only secondary but, moreover, a consequence of what they perceived to be unwarranted ill-treatment toward them by particular people in their lives. In this respect, they were angry victims.

In all cases their murder victims were being punished for something they did or something they represented to their killer. Blaming others for their misdeeds is one of the dynamics that shapes their experience of entitlement. Victims were seen as deserving of what they got. One subject described his killings as being "on a revenge trip." He explained his series of murders as displaced attempts to kill his first girlfriend – who jilted him. He explained the murders as the result of his anger at her for having humiliated him. "They were paying for her sins."

It should be noted that it is not that these men lacked a basic moral code, for each of them provided many instances of situations in which they believed someone else had acted wrongly toward someone (not necessarily themselves). Subjects did appear to have a set of values regarding appropriate and acceptable behaviors. In each case, however, they applied these rules differentially to themselves. One subject spoke about experiences he had while living in a foster home after his parents had relinquished their responsibility for him, telling him that they could no longer "handle" him. He was sent to a home in which the male head of the household was molesting one of the female foster children. The subject related:

> The foster parents were pillars of society and all this stuff, but I caught the step-father having sex with the stepdaughter. I was really religious and it really turned me right off because these people would sit in the front pew of the Lutheran church with the Assistant Mayor and the Police Chief. And these people would come home and do this to their kids. So it really turned me off of religion – and everything.

Then, incredibly, he ended the discussion on this matter with the calm disclosure –in fact boasting about it– "I blackmailed him for $20 a day – to go to the [fair]." This subject seemed to have no sense that while he had recognized what his foster father did was wrong, his own behavior –taking opportunistic advantage of the situation by blackmailing the foster father– attached culpability to him, as well. It was as if what he did was not subject to the same kinds of rules or judgments that he has applied to others.

This kind of thinking, reminiscent of Yochelson and Samenow's (1976) "thinking errors" revealed itself over and over again with all five subjects. It was not that these men failed to understand that what they did was wrong in the eyes of society. Nor was it that they lacked any personal moral code. It was rather that what they did was evaluated according to an individuated – and bifurcated– set of rules: one for them and one for everyone else. The fact that subjects believed they had an "acceptable" motive for some misdeed – meaning it was something they needed to do for themselves– served as its justification. Such a "biased" personal code of values would facilitate the experience of entitlement, enabling them to engage in behaviors that they would not tolerate in others.

In relating the accounts of his killings, each subject manifested an ability to cognitively empathize with his victims but appeared to lack any degree of emotional empathy. Typical in this regard was a subject who was asked about his victims' "state" when they were being killed. Regarding the second victim he related, "Don't think about her. Never have. Never had any regrets at all. She was in an alcoholic stupor anyway. I don't think she'd be rational anyway. I knew she was aware she was getting hurt. I knew that." Like each of the other subjects, he knew on one level that he was hurting his victim – indeed he was motivated by that knowledge. He did not, however, appear to attach any emotional meaning to that fact. He seemed incapable of relating to their terror. The entitlement he felt was unencumbered by emotionally identifying with those he harmed. Perhaps another subject said it best: "I had too much anger. There was no room for any feelings for her."

6.2. Control/Empowerment

As subjects discussed their series of murders a second theme emerged which appeared to be a critical factor in the way they experienced their crimes. All five serial murderers related that the killings empowered them – gave them an undeniable sense of control, albeit fleeting. The theme of empowerment was also expressed in their fantasies. Each subject talked about the major role fantasy has played throughout his life – before and during his incarceration. Fantasy involves the creation of an "other" reality. Its predominance throughout the lives of these subjects may be accounted for by the nature of any fantasy: It confers the experience of complete control – over others and over one's own destiny. Desired outcomes are virtually assured. Real-world exigencies do not intrude upon the experience of success and personal gratification, making fantasies especially seductive. As one subject remarked, however,

> A lot of time you were just satisfied with the fantasy of killing. So you didn't need to go through with killing. That will carry you, sustain you. But sometimes the urge gets so strong that the fantasy isn't enough. And after you kill your fantasy is even better – until it isn't good enough again. Like a vicious circle or something.

Fantasies enabled subjects to experience themselves as "more than they were." It seems, however, that the actual image they had of themselves as powerless and inconsequential remained within the peripheral vision of their mind's eye and threatened to expose their insecurity. Enacting the fantasy – actualization of the fantasized self– challenged the credibility, and therefore authenticity, of the image of the self as powerless. Hence the potency of enacting the fantasy. Doing so transformed the offender into a person of consequence, bestowing a tremendous measure of power. ("Not everyone can do what I did.")

One of the murderers detailed his four killings and explained that with "the sex, there was a definite feeling of using the person. Physically using – and abusing– her. My penis was a weapon. The rape part of the assault was part of the effort to degrade and humiliate. It wasn't like sexual gratification. It was diminishing her by taking what I wanted. It was domination." Since the sexual violation of his victims included biting their breasts, the subject's choice of the word "domination" here –in the context of his descriptions of "destroying" his victims– suggests that what he experienced as "domination" might be better understood as "abomination."

Like the other subjects, this serial murderer felt excited by the power he had over his victims as he killed them, taking away from them any control he felt they (or what they represented to him) had over him – over his emotions. Killing became a way to relieve himself of the burden of the "knowledge" (read, experience) of his impotence.

6.3. Vitality

As subjects recalled their murders another aspect of the killing experience emerged – not unrelated to control but also not the same. Killing made them feel alive; experienced as an euphoric "high" or a violent anger that they acted out giving them great pleasure. This was followed by a welcomed state of calm; a sense of relief. They all described being unable to sustain these feelings after a murder and found themselves becoming increasingly restless and easily agitated – feelings that were numbed with alcohol, displaced by fantasies, and ultimately (temporarily) dispatched by killing again.

> I was so afraid of losing control. The tensions, the pressure, didn't go away. I would push it down and down until I couldn't push it down anymore – it blew up. It came out. The only reason I realized it was because of the lack of pressure I felt right after the murders. A complete feeling of drain. I realized how much I got out to empty all of that, so how much I must have been carrying. And for a few days afterward I would still feel more relaxed and normal. But that was a short-lived feeling. Very quickly the feeling of the pressure was there again – which was actually the more normal state for me. So while I thought that I was becoming more normalized, I was actually becoming dangerous again.

Some subjects claimed that they frequently used alcohol as a way of coping with the depressed and destructive feelings they had regarding their lives. But when their sense of self was directly threatened, they concentrated their energies as protection against their "assailants." The result was that one subject killed females who had "reduced him [through humiliation] to nothing," and another killed in order to guard against being "taken over by homosexuality" at all costs. In both these cases subjects reported that the killings temporarily relieved them of their dread of "being nothing" or of "losing himself." For the remaining three subjects killing seems to have provided a kind of excitement that went beyond anything they had previously experienced in their lives –essentially elevating them to an experience of themselves as omnipotent– in contrast with an otherwise "powerless" existence. On some level the killings provided each subject with a sense of being somebody of consequence – in marked contrast with the way he generally experienced himself, in childhood and as an adult. The killings transformed him into someone with the power of life over death – an experience that was life-affirming. For all five subjects, killing preserved or heightened their experiences of vitality. The murders prompted a kind of experiential transcendence – from helpless victim to omnipotent killer.

The subjects in this study were told that although results of the interviews with them may be published, their names would not be disclosed. In all cases subjects immediately responded that they had no problem with the use of their names. The need for celebrity, an equivalent of vitality, was apparent. As one subject said of his killings, "They made me famous." His murders established him in society –and in history– albeit in infamy.

Since sex as a life-equivalent is generally associated with vitality, the sexualization of aggression is frequently observed in fantasies of serial murderers. In recalling his murders, one of the serial killers had distinct memories of the anger he felt while at the same time being intensely sexually aroused as he was killing his victims. "I feel most alive when I'm angry. And if I'm more uptight my sex drive gets stronger. Both these feelings [anger and sexual arousal] were there when I killed. I felt more alive when I was destroying and humiliating my victims." His revelation that destroying (by killing) made him feel complete suggests that he otherwise had a sense of himself as diminished or not intact. Like the other subjects his impulse to destroy seems predicated on a need to preserve his self. He presented what he thought was the main driving force behind his murders:

> The feeling I've always had is to destroy. Destroy in the sense of totally obliterate – more than kill. Destroy involves, to me, much more than just killing – which is very quick. . . .There's something in me that wanted to end up with the victim dead – and beyond that – to destroy her. . . .The urge to destroy was the key drive. . . .I learned what to do to get a release, like an addiction. I needed to destroy to feel complete.

In contrast with most people whose experience of vitality as it relates to sex derives from the sense of "I come therefore I am," for these serial murderers affirmation of their being required that they kill. One subject described the strength of his urge to kill as follows:

> I remember while strangling the victims telling myself to open my hands – to stop doing this. It's like having a ball thrown at you and it hits you. I could not move. A very large part of me wanted to destroy and the rational side of me could not stop it. It was overpowering. My emotional side was in charge.

The interviews with these men revealed that serial murderers appear to be driven by the same kinds of motive forces experienced by other people; however their sense of entitlement, need for empowerment, and quest for vitality take them far beyond the boundaries that contain the rest of us.

7. CONCLUDING REMARKS

The three themes that so dominated subjects' discussion of their murders – entitlement, empowerment, and vitality– appeared to structure their experiences of killing in the sense that they were what made the repeated killings meaningful to them. This research suggests that serial murderers can be distinguished from others by the way they experience entitlement, empowerment, and vitality. The importance of these themes in their killings derives from the emotional meaning these men attached to their lived experiences with these themes in other aspects of their lives.

The five subjects in this study presented formative histories in which they experienced themselves as essentially impotent: as victims of other people and circumstance; as individuals without control in their own lives; and as individuals lacking an inherent sense of vitality. In some instances there were situations that triggered emotional memories of earlier experiences in their lives. The feelings associated with their formative experiences seem to have provided an emotional blueprint to which later life experiences were compared. It was the emotional meaning of these experiences that appeared to activate and direct their violent behaviors.

The interviews also served to reveal a striking trait apparent in all five subjects. It is as if these men essentially perceived the world in terms of "black or white" and were lacking in the capacity to "see" (i.e., experience) the world in color.[5] They appeared unable to discern complexity and instead reduced the world to dimensional polarities. For example, things tend to be good or bad. One is right or wrong. Such constrained vision of the world narrows one's experiences, facilitating the kind of skewed emotional meanings that these subjects seemed to link with their experiences. The emotional component of subjects' experiences seemed to delineate and, indeed, determine their meaning and constitute a powerful motivating force in their killings. This observation is consistent with psychophysiological measures of psychopaths under laboratory conditions. Research suggests that (criminal) psychopaths are aberrant in the terms of their processing of emotional information as compared with non-psychopaths (Williamson, Harpur & Hare, 1991) and nonpsychopathic offenders (Christianson, Forth, Hare, Strachan, Lidberg & Thorell, 1996). To the extent psychopaths extract information from their emotional experiences differently than do others, aberrations in their behavioral responses to emotional situations (and to triggered emotional memories) may be understood.

Again, the three themes that dominated descriptions of the killing experiences of the five subjects are not themes that would distinguish these men as serial killers. Most people have feelings of entitlement that can motivate them to behave assertively if not aggressively when they believe they have been denied what is their due. Most people will tend to behave in ways that give them a greater sense of control in their lives. And most people have a need to feel they have potency in the world – that they are of some consequence. This research does suggest, however, that while serial murderers are motivated by the same kinds of forces that motivate the rest of us, for them these same forces are exaggerated and distorted. The extent to which aspects of the three themes permeate the experiences of their lives – not only their killings– suggests that they are instrumental –if not fundamental– to the process by which they experience themselves and organize their lives.

For all subjects the killings served as a means to sustain themselves – literally by disabling victims from identifying them, or by taking away the power that their victims were perceived to have over them. It is as if the killings were a way to reconstitute or preserve themselves in the face of an impending doom. For each subject the series of murders seemed to be a way to reconstitute a fragmenting self into a more integrated whole. The threat of "being nobody," experienced in different ways by different subjects –and coupled with the rage they felt at this– not only enabled them to kill but impelled them to do what they did. While there is not a single indication that any of the victims of these men presented an actual threat to their physical being – all but one of them killed when they felt threatened by people or circumstances they feared had the power to diminish them. And in the remaining case the killing made him feel like he was "somebody" – which may speak to the same threat but on a more superficial level.

In killing, the serial murderer is moved from the experience of himself as reactive object to proactive agent – victim becoming victimizer. The one without power overcomes that which will otherwise diminish him. Killing is a matter of controlling the threat, controlling the source of power that threatens his own. In the end what appears outwardly to be offensive behavior is essentially defensive. And the violence itself is reinforced, indelibly linked to his experience of vitality. On some level for all subjects, killing meant living – it became the means to experience a viable sense of themselves in the world. Untoward factors in his formative development may not only shape him but can also revisit him in adulthood in the form of emotional memories with tremendous motive power.

When these men felt emotional pain or anger or fear they generally did one of two things: they numbed or displaced these feelings with drugs or alcohol, or they expressed them with an intensity and in a manner far in excess of acceptable limits. Once these men killed they learned they could alleviate their dis-ease through acts of murder. After killing for the first time and experiencing the release from their discomforting feelings –temporarily replaced by experiencing themselves as powerful and alive, reinforcing their sense of entitlement– killing became the way to feel better. More than merely making the bad feelings go away, killing became the way to make these men feel good, and in so doing, limited –if not precluded– their personal growth. Individually, each murder sustained them in the moment; collectively, the series of murders fashioned a purpose for their lives. They became, as it were, "stuck" in their violence. Each one of them stated that he would not have stopped killing had he not been caught.

What was most apparent from this research is that subjects appeared to attach emotional meanings to their experiences that were exaggerated or skewed as compared with the way other people experience similar situations. This was immediately apparent when subjects used words that suggested common experiences but upon further probing were found to have substantially different meanings for them than is generally connoted by those particular words. It is as if these subjects were using "emotional homonyms" – words that sounded the same but had different emotional meanings for them, recalling, as an example, the use of the word "angry" by one subject to describe his actual experience of "being empty." This observation points to the particular value of the phenomenological method, aimed as it is at revealing an individual's lived-meaning of the world, it does not assume an understanding but rather works at developing it – using the terms of meaning constructed by the subject.

The atypical use of language by the serial killers in this study may be explained by findings of psychophysiological research regarding psychopaths, leaving us with important questions about the extent to which the etiology of psychopathy overlaps with that of serial murder; as well as questions about whether structures of the brain that ordinarily impart emotionality to experience –and which determine motivation– are the primary site of dysfunction in the serial killer. In raising these questions, this paper moves us closer to the kind of interdisciplinary orientation that is needed to more comprehensively understand serial murder.

Murder, in its most fundamental aspect, is about self-preservation. How it is committed is largely a matter of gender; but why it is committed is a function of the human condition.

And so, too, for serial killing. The outward facts of serial killings may serve to mask more substantive similarities between serial killers and the rest of us. We are not, it would seem, distinguished by the nature of our being but rather by the meanings we create from our respective lived-experiences.

The very existence of the serial murderer shatters our image of what constitutes being human. In this sense, the predatory killings of serial killers convict us all, revealing the depths of man's inhumanity.

NOTES

[1] There is no consensus among or between scholars and law enforcement agents as to what constitutes serial murder. A number of articles have been devoted to this issue. [See, for example, Keeney & Heide (1995) and Egger (1990).] This work defines serial murder as the killing of three or more people (not associated with a political or occupational role) over a period of time by the same person(s).

[2] Imre Horvath. (Producer). (1984). Rainbow Broadcasting Company.

[3] In referring to serial murderers, except where the discussion involves female killers specifically, masculine pronouns are used in this paper to facilitate flow of the document. While most known serial murderers are male, approximately 15 percent of serial murderers are female. Thus the reader is cautioned against thinking of serial murder as an exclusively male phenomenon.

[4] Tom Roberts (Executive Producer). (1995). "Minds to Crime." A Quality Time Production for Channel Four in association with The Learning Channel.

[5] Each subject revealed this "black or white" perspective of the world in many ways. Examples are numerous. As one of the killers related, "If people love me I love them back with all I got. But when I hate, I hate with a ferocity of Satan. And, you can either be my friend or my enemy – there's no in between." Another subject talked about power as the most important aspect of a person's life: "You either have it or you don't." SUBJECT #1 spoke of people as "either hurtful or hurt." Such examples reflect a rigidity on the part of these subjects in terms of the personal model of the world they construct for themselves. While they appear to organize their experience of the world in accordance with the same dimensions that other people use (e.g., being powerful – being impotent; being loved – being unloved; being a victim – being a victimizer) the manner in which they apply these dimensions appears to be decidedly polarized.

REFERENCES

Bailey, K. G. (1987): *Human paleopsychology: applications to aggression and pathological processes*, Hillsdale N.J., Lawrence Erlbaum Associates.

Christianson, S-A; Forth, A. E.; Hare, R. D.; Strachan, C.; Lidberg, L. & Thorell, L-H. (1996): "Remembering details of emotional events: A comparison between psychopathic and nonpsychopathic offenders", *Personality and Individual Differences*, 20(4), pp. 437-443.

Dietz, P. E. (1986): "Mass, serial and sensational homicides", *Bulletin of the New York Academy of Medicine*, 62(5), pp. 477-490.

Egger, S. A. (1990): "Serial murder: a synthesis of literature and research", in S. A. Egger (ed.), *Serial murder: an elusive phenomenon*, New York, Praeger.

Hare, R. D. (1993): *Without conscience: the disturbing world of the psychopaths among us*, New York, Pocket Books.

Hare, R. D. (1970): *Psychopathy: theory and research*, New York, John Wiley & Sons.

Keeney, B. T. & Heide, K. M. (1995): "Serial murder: a more accurate and inclusive definition", *International Journal of Offender Therapy and Comparative Criminology*, 39(4), pp. 299-306.

Money, J. (1990): "Forensic sexology: Paraphilic serial rape (blastophilia) and lust murder (erotophonophilia)", *American Journal of Psychotherapy* XLIV(1), pp. 26-36.

Raine, A. (1994): "Selective reductions in prefrontal glucose metabolism in murderers", *Society of Biological Psychiatry*, 36, pp. 365-373.

Raine, A. (1993): *The psychopathology of crime: criminal behavior as a clinical disorder*, New York, Academic Press.

Reeve, J. (1992): *Understanding motivation and emotion*, New York, Harcourt Brace Jovanovich College Publishers.

Skrapec, C. A. (1997): *Serial murder: Motive and meaning*, Dissertation Abstracts International, (University Microfilms No. 9808004).

Skrapec, C. A. (1996): "The sexual component of serial murder", in T. O'Reilly-Fleming (ed.), *Serial & mass murder: theory, research and policy*, Toronto, Canadian Scholars Press.

Skrapec, C. A. (1994): "The female serial killer: an evolving criminality", in H. Birch (ed.), *Moving targets: women, murder and representation*, Berkeley, University of California Press.

Williamson, S.; Harpur, J. & Hare, R. D. (1991): "Abnormal processing of affective words by psychopaths", *Psychophysiology*, 28(3), pp. 260-273.

Wrangham, R. & Peterson, D. (1996): *Demonic males: apes and the origins of human violence*, New York, Mariner Books.

Yochelson, S. & Samenow, S. E. (1976): *The criminal personality: volume I: a profile for change*, New York, Jason Aronson.

Chapter 7

PSYCHOPATHY, SADISM AND SERIAL KILLING

David J. Cooke
Douglas Inch Centre and Glasgow Caledonian University, Scotland, UK

1. PSYCHOPATHY, SADISM AND SERIAL KILLING

Like all complex human behavior serial killing is underpinned by a skein of interrelated and interacting processes; biological, social and psychological processes (Raine, 1993; Skrapec, this volume). Within the domain of personality disorder the two forms of disorder which have been most frequently implicated are psychopathy and sadistic personality disorder (SPD). It is not surprising that these disorders have been implicated as both entail predispositions to violence in general, and instrumental violence in particular (Cornell et al., 1995; Millon & Davis, 1996). These disorders are important not only because they can provide the motive to engage in serial killing –e.g., the need to dominate and humiliate– but also, they entail the absence of characteristics that would act as barriers to cruel and demeaning behavior –lack of empathy, shallow affect and callousness.

In terms of empirical understanding the two disorders could not be more different. Psychopathy is the most widely researched personality disorder, and in recent years an extensive network of laboratory, clinical and forensic evidence has demonstrated the validity and utility of the construct (e.g., Cooke, Forth, & Hare, 1998; Hare, 1996; Millon, 1981). By way of sharp contrast, there is little agreement about the defining features of SPD; there is little evidence to support the utility or validity of the construct.

In this chapter, I will briefly review the relevance of psychopathy to serial killing, I will then examine the evidence for the utility of the construct of SPD and explore the available evidence regarding the validity of this construct.

Violence and Psychopathy, edited by Raine & Sanmartin,
Kluwer Academic/Plenum Publishers, New York, 2001.

2. RECENT RESEARCH ON THE NATURE OF PSYCHOPATHY

The development of the Psychopathy Checklist - Revised (PCL-R; Hare, 1991) has provided a clear and stable operationalisation of psychopathy, this has lead to an impressive array of evidence supporting the validity of the construct (See Hare, Patrick, Raine this volume and Cooke, Forth, & Hare, 1998). I do not intend to repeat what has been so admirably covered elsewhere in this volume, however, I will briefly indicate how new psychometric analyses of criteria for psychopathy may enhance our understanding of the role of this disorder in relation to serial killing.

Psychopathy is a form of personality disorder characterized by distinct interpersonal, affective and behavioral features (Cleckley, 1976; Hare, 1970; 1991). Within the interpersonal domain, psychopaths are arrogant, grandiose, superficially charming; they lie easily and manipulate others. Within the affective domain they lack the capacity to experience emotion, for example, they lack guilt and the capacity to feel empathy. Within the behavioral domain they are irresponsible, impulsive, they lack goals and are parasitic in relation to others.

Brief consideration of these three domains indicates that these symptoms have salience for serial killing. The interpersonal skills necessary to charm, con and manipulate others may assist the psychopath to acquire victims. The cases of Ted Bundy illustrates this point admirably: he has been described as an articulate, educated, suave and handsome man. His modus operandi was to put his arm in a sling and pretend to have a broken arm, he would ask his potential victim to assist him to put his groceries in his car; once his victim was in the car, he would rip off his sling and trap her.

The affective deficits of an inability to feel guilt or experience empathy means that the psychopath can engage in the humiliation and torture of victims without experiencing the inhibiting effects of distress. The salience of this deficit is perhaps most evident amongst the group of serial killers who engage in the torture of their victims, examples, would include Ian Brady and Fred West in England, Chikatilo in Russia and John Wayne Gacy in the United States.

Perhaps the behavioral domain of psychopathy is of somewhat lesser relevance to serial killing. On the one hand, the tendency to reckless behavior –behavior that disregards the rights and interests of others– may increase the likelihood that an individual will engage in this type of behavior, on the other hand, the impulsivity and inability to plan ahead would inhibit the successful serial killer. Planning is important for certain forms of serial killing. One facet of the behavioral domain is proneness to boredom, in some case this characteristic may come into play. Stone (1998) indicated that Loeb and his friends –wealthy, bored and sensation-seeking adolescents– killed a young boy in order to add spice to their monotonous life.

Until recently there has been a conflict between the clinical tradition that has emphasized these three distinct, but interrelated domains of symptoms, and the empirical tradition that has emphasized two distinct, yet correlated, factors (Harpur, Hakstian, & Hare, 1988). In some recent analysis my colleague Chistine Michie and I have sought to refine and clarify the link between the clinical and empirical traditions. Using confirmatory analysis of over 3000 cases and 3 measures of psychopathy we have developed a 3-factor model of psychopathy (Cooke & Michie, 1999a). Using both statistical criteria derived from item response analyses (Cooke & Michie, 1997; Cooke & Michie, 1999b, Cooke, Michie, Hart, & Hare, 1998), and theoretical consideration, we developed a hierarchical structural model using 13 of the PCL-R items.

Within this model, a superordinate factor, which we term psychopathy, is underpinned by three distinct but related first order factors. The first factor measures interpersonal style. It is defined by the PCL-R items *glibness and superficial charm, grandiose sense of self-worth, pathological lying* and *conning/manipulative*. We have called this factor Arrogant and Deceitful Interpersonal Style. Factor two represents an affective factor being specified by the PCL-R items *shallow affect, callous/lack of empathy, lack of remorse or guilt* and *failure to accept responsibility*. We have called this factor Deficient Affective Experience. Factor three represents a behavioral factor specified by *need for stimulation/proneness to boredom, impulsivity, irresponsibility, parasitic lifestyle* and *lack of realistic, long term goals*. We have called this factor Impulsive and Irresponsible Behavioral Style. Given that all these first order factor contribute to a higher order factor, and this superordinate factor shows high factor saturation, we consider that this higher order factor can be defined as psychopathy. This model not only fitted the data well but also was cross-validated across culture and across methods for measuring psychopathy.

It will be noted that we only used 13 of the 20 PCL-R items in this model. This is for both statistical and theoretical reasons. Statistically, the deleted items contributed very little information to the measurement of the underlying trait. Removing seven of the 20 items has the conceptual advantage that it removes items that could add circularity to the argument that psychopathy influences offending; the items to do with offending, e.g., early behavioral problems, juvenile delinquency, criminal versatility were removed from the model.

3. PSYCHOPATHY AND SERIAL KILLING

Stone (1998) has provided the most systematic study of the relationship between serial killing and psychopathy. In a novel approach he reviewed 279 "true crime" biographies of murderers. While these cannot be regarded as a systematic sample of murderers as a whole, they do provide accounts of the more extreme forms of homicidal behavior. It is noteworthy that 61 out of the 63 male serial killers in Stone's sample met PCL-R criteria for psychopathy. It would be interesting to know what PCL-R profiles these individuals displayed in relation to the 3 factors of psychopathy outlined above: are the majority high on factor one and factor two, and low on the Impulsive and Irresponsible Behavioral Style factor? It would appear, therefore, from the limited systematic evidence that psychopathy is a frequent feature of serial killing and should be taken into account when we try to understand this growing phenomenon.

Given that psychopathy has been explored in detail in this volume, I will now turn to that more elusive personality disorder, SPD. I will begin by placing it in historical context before examining the defining features of the disorder in some detail.

4. SADISTIC PERSONALITY DISORDER

Sadistic Personality Disorder entails cruel, demeaning and aggressive interactions with other people. By definition SPD starts early in life, it is long lasting and pervades an individual's interactions with others at school, work, in social contexts and within family relationships. The term 'sadism' was coined by Krafft-Ebing (1898) originally to describe fantasies and behavior focused on inflicting pain during sexual interactions. Krafft-Ebing drew on the writings of the 18th-century author, the Marquis de Sade, and indicated that the sadist experiences sexual arousal by exercising control and dominance, pain and humiliation on the object of their desire.

Since Krafft-Ebing's original description, the construct of SPD has broadened to embrace a wide range of personality traits and interpersonal behaviors that affect all social encounters not merely sexual encounters. Recent clinical descriptions suggests that the features of the disorder are diverse and wide ranging – and as with psychopathy, they span the behavioral, the interpersonal, the cognitive and the affective domains (Fiester & Gay, 1991, 1995; Millon & Davies, 1996).

At the behavioral level, sadistic individuals have poor behavioral controls – they are irritable and flare up easily in response to minor frustrations. Sadistic individuals use a wide range of behaviors, from the hostile glance to severe physical punishment, in order to exercise control. Although they may engage in expressive violence – violence underpinned by emotions such as anger and frustration – much of their violence is instrumental, its purpose being to intimidate and control, and thereby, obtain gratification.

At the interpersonal level, these individuals are abrasive particularly towards those whom they perceive as their inferiors. The more socially adept sadist may achieve satisfaction and control by derisive social comments and cutting remarks, others may achieve the same ends in a more overtly hostile manner, by threatening, coercing or the intimidation of others. They may exercise inappropriate control over others, the sadistic father may forbid his daughter to attend a late night disco, the sadistic husband may prevent his wife meeting with friends, while the sadistic boss may bully and exploit a subordinate (Millon & Davies, 1996). It is a frequent feature in populations of spousal assaulters (Hart, Dutton, & Newlove, 1993).

At the cognitive level sadistic individuals are frequently rigid and dogmatic; their values are authoritarian and intolerant, for example, they may construe out-groups as being devoid of any value, racism and prejudice is clearly evident. Feister & Gay (1995) reported that they often attribute malevolent intent to the behavior of others and are over sensitive to what they construe as the derisive behavior of others. They may have unusual interests. Brittain (1970) in his classic clinical account of the sadistic murderer, argued that their interests may include concentration camps, atrocities, black magic, sexual perversions, toxicology, crime and criminals, murders and murderers. Many sadists will be familiar with the writings of De Sade, the more sophisticated with the writings of Nietzsche.

At the affective level, the sadist shares many of the critical features of the psychopath: they lack remorse for their controlling and exploitative behavior, they do not experience shame or guilt, and they are unable to empathize with their victims. They are cold hearted.

It is important to emphasize that these characteristics are high-order personality constructs and can be expressed in differing ways in differing contexts. Perhaps the most obvious form is the tyrannical sadist who abuses, intimidates and humiliates his victim in front of their work colleagues; he obtains pleasure from the psychic pain and distress of those whom he subjugates. The sadist may seek and achieve social positions that allows the exercising of control and the opportunity to mete out punishment in socially sanctioned roles. Examples would include the judge who metes out punishment of a cruel and unusual severity, the army sergeant who brutalizes the new recruit, and the psychiatrist who misuses mental health legislation to incarcerate a patient.

5. THE NATURE OF SADISTIC PERSONALITY DISORDER

The concept of SPD can be seen to have emerged from constructs in the psychological, psychiatric and psychoanalytic traditions (Widiger, Frances, Spitzer & Williams, 1988). Millon (1981) has argued cogently that there is a need for systematic description to describe those individuals whose underlying temperament is domineering, intimidating, malicious and hostile, who are short-tempered, and who engage in physically cruel behavior. Widiger and Trull (1994) argued that these traits are not well described by criteria for ASPD nor criteria for psychopathy (Hare, 1991). For example, only one PCL-R item is directly focused on aggressive behavior: *poor behavioral controls* is concerned primarily with disproportionately aggressive and violent responses to frustration, failure or disputes. Thus, it is technically possible for an individual to be psychopathic without displaying this characteristic – indeed, in the new three factor formulation of the disorder poor behavioral controls does not contribute to the definition of psychopathy (Cooke & Michie, 199b).

An attempt was made to systemize the description of the disorder by introducing criteria for SPD in appendix A of DSM-III-R, "Proposed Diagnostic Categories Needing Further Study" (American Psychiatric Association, 1987): These criteria are included here as they represent the criteria set for which there is most, albeit limited, empirical data.

Diagnostic Criteria for Sadistic Personality Disorder (433)

A. A pervasive pattern of cruel, demeaning, and aggressive behavior, beginning by early adulthood, as indicated by the repeated occurrence of at least four of the following:

(1) has used physical cruelty or violence for the purpose of establishing dominance in a relationship (not merely to achieve some noninterpersonal goal, such as striking someone in order to rob him or her)
(2) humiliates or demeans people in the presence of others
(3) has treated or disciplined someone under his or her controlled unusually harshly, e.g., a child, student, prisoner, or patient
(4) is amused by, or takes pleasure in, the psychological or physical suffering of others (including animals)
(5) has lied for the purpose of harming or inflicting pain on others (not merely to achieve some other goal)
(6) gets other people to do what he or she wants by frightening them (through intimidation or even terror)
(7) restricts the autonomy of people with whom he or she has a close relationship, e.g., will not let spouse leave the house unaccompanied or permit teen-age daughter to attend social functions
(8) is fascinated by violence, weapons, martial arts, injury, or torture

B. The behavior in A has not been directed towards only one person (e.g., spouse, one child) and has not been şolely for the purpose of sexual arousal (as in Sexual Sadism).

Table 1. Diagnostic Criteria for Sadistic Personality Disorder

Examination of these criteria reveals conceptual, if not necessarily empirical, coherence in the first 7 features of criterion A – these features all relate to different methods for gaining power and control over others. There is an unfortunate emphasize on the behavioral rather than the affective and cognitive components of the disorder: perhaps this reflects the mistaken belief that clinicians are unable to assess these domains reliably. This deficit in the definition of SPD parallels the deficit found in the definition of ASPD (Hart & Hare, 1995).

In a recent study, Berger, Berner, Bolterauer, Gutierrez, and Berger (1999) examined the interrelationships between the DSM-III SPD criteria and other DSM personality features in a sample of 70 sex offenders (27 child molesters, 33 rapists, and 10 murderers). What is noteworthy about their study is that they carried out a factor analysis on a range of personality disorder characteristics, they found a distinct factor specified by the SPD criteria, together with two ASPD criteria relating to violence and cruelty. Although carried out on a limited sample size, this analysis provides some evidence that SPD criteria may form a coherent syndrome, not in the sense of a diagnostic group, but rather in the sense of a group of symptoms that occur together and can be distinguished from other syndromes.

Given that the systematic description of this disorder is fairly recent, the disorder is comparative rare, and perhaps, the difficulty inherent in obtaining reliable information about the critical features: it is not surprising that the literature available regarding the validity of the construct and the prevalence, comorbidity and demographic distribution is extremely limited. I will now considered this limited evidence.

6. PREVALENCE

Fiester and Gay (1995) provide a valuable summary of what is known about this disorder. Less than ten empirical studies are apparent in the literature (3 of which are unpublished and are quoted in Fiester & Gay, 1995): they provide some limited information about the prevalence of SPD in clinical and forensic populations. A postal survey of forensic psychiatrists, found that around 2.5% of forensic psychiatric cases evaluated by their respondents in the previous year met the criteria for SPD. Unfortunately, it is difficult to generalize from this postal survey as the response rate was only 20%. In a sample of 176 outpatients attending a mental health clinic in rural Georgia, USA, it was found that 8% of the sample met DSM-IIIR criteria for SPD. Gay (1989) found that approximately 5% met the diagnostic criteria for SPD in a sample of 235 adults who had been accused of child abuse. The unpublished data reported by Fiester and Gay (1995) may suggest greater variance in prevalence. Freiman and Widiger (1989) assessed a sample of 50 psychiatric hospital inpatients using the Personality Interview Questionnaire-II; a substantial number, 18% of this sample were diagnosed as having SPD.

Not surprisingly, the prevalence of SPD among serial killers is extremely high. Stone (1998) used biographical data to obtain DSM-III-R and DSM-IV diagnoses for 79 male serial killers. He reported that 90% of the sample met the DSM-III-R criteria for SPD. Other personality disorders in the sample with high prevalence were antisocial (81%), narcissistic (61%) and schizoid (48%) personality disorder. Berger et al. (1999) in their study of sex offenders found 27.2% of the sample of 70 participants met the diagnostic criteria for SPD. This was consistent with previous findings on a smaller sample of sex offenders (n=30) published by the same authors (Berner, Berger, Gutierrez, Jordan, & Berger, 1992). Hart et al. (1993) found that 26.5% of a small sample (n=34) of wife assaulters met the criteria for SPD.

As might be expected the prevalence of the disorder appears to be lower amongst non-offender populations. Millon and Tringone (1989) found that the prevalence of SPD in a sample of outpatients was only 3%.

Thus, a review of the literature indicates that our systematic knowledge about the prevalence of SPD is extremely limited. A number of factors –the paucity of studies, the inadequacy of sample size and sampling procedures, the variation in diagnostic procedures adopted– mitigate against the provision of any accurate estimate of the prevalence of this disorder. Both the clinical literature and the limited empirical literature available suggest that SPD is primarily a disorder of males (Freiman & Widiger, 1989; Gay, 1989; Spitzer, Fiester, Gay & Pfohl, 1991); no research has examined whether this difference could in part be attributed to gender bias in the individual diagnostic criteria (cf. Hartung & Widiger, 1998).

7. COMORBIDITY OF SADISTIC PERSONALITY DISORDER WITH OTHER PERSONALITY DISORDERS

The absence of convincing and reliable prevalence data for this disorder means that it is inappropriate to provide quantitative estimates of the degree of comorbidity with other Axis II disorders. At a descriptive level the available studies imply that there will be comorbidity between SPD and both APSD and Narcissistic PD (Freiman & Widiger, 1989; Gay, 1989; Spitzer, Fiester, Gay & Pfohl, 1991). Fiester and Gay (1995) indicated that the high comorbidity of SPD with other disorders may call into question the discreteness of the category: this of course is not peculiar to SPD.

With regard to psychopathy, it is likely that SPD will demonstrate an asymmetric relationship with psychopathy; most sadists are likely to show significant psychopathic traits while not all psychopaths will necessarily display traits of SPD. I am not aware of any data that addresses this issue directly in general populations or in forensic samples. However, in Stone's (1998) biographical analysis of serial killers, described above, the prevalence of both SPD and psychopathy (as measured by PCL-R cutoff of 25) was about 90%, suggesting that the comorbidity of the two disorders in this unusual sample was very high.

8. PROBLEMS IN THE ASSESSMENT OF SADISTIC PERSONALITY DISORDER

The nature of the defining characteristic of the disorder are such that those being assessed are likely to deny or minimize the presence of these characteristics. It is difficult to get patients to admit to cruel, demeaning and aggressive behavior, particularly when the demand characteristics of the situation –for example, a risk assessment for court– will militate against the patient being open (Dietz, Hazelwood, & Warren, 1990). Access to considerable collateral data is necessary to ensure valid evaluation. The SPD criteria are essentially behaviorally based, and in particular, fail to tap the cognitive or affective characteristics that clinical descriptions of the disorder emphasize. Extensive research with the PCL-R demonstrates that it is possible for clinicians to assess related constructs in a reliable and valid manner, and thus, the argument that clinicians are inherent incapable of achieving adequate assessments of these domains cannot be used as a valid argument (Hare, 1991). More comprehensive and sophisticated criteria are required for SPD if our understanding of this disorder is to progress.

9. THE ABSENCE OF OFFICIALLY RECOGNIZED CRITERIA FOR SADISTIC PERSONALITY DISORDER

From the researcher's perspective the position has deteriorated because no officially sanctioned criteria for the disorder are now available. SPD criteria were included in appendix A of DSM-III-R, "Proposed Diagnostic Categories Needing Further Study" (American Psychological Association, 1987). The criteria were included in response to a demand from clinicians who observed SPD amongst spousal assaulters and child abusers (Widiger, 1995). The intention underpinning the inclusion of SPD was not to establish the disorder as an officially sanctioned disorder, but perhaps surprisingly, in order to stimulate more research directed at clarifying whether SPD should be recognized as a distinct disorder (Widiger, 1995). A range of considerations influenced the deletion of the disorder from DSM-IV (American Psychological Association, 1994). The primary consideration was the lack of a coherent body of research concerning the validity and utility of the concept (Widiger, 1995). In addition, it was thought that enshrining the disorder in DSM-IV – thereby providing it with official status – could lead to the misuse of the diagnosis in forensic settings. It was envisaged that those suffering from the SPD might use the diagnosis in attempts to mitigate their responsibility for their violence against women and against children (Feister & Gay, 1989). Stone expounded the line of thinking: "Inclusion of SPD might, in other words, lead to the 'medicalization of evil deeds' – a step on the way to trivializing their impact and inadvertently sanitizing them by offering the excuse that they were the result of an 'illness'" (Stone, 1998, p. 347). Indeed, 76% of the respondents to a survey of forensic psychiatrists held that the diagnosis had considerable potential for abuse (Spitzer, Fiester, Gay & Pfohl, 1991).

Despite these arguments, it has been contended forcefully that the deletion of the SPD from the nomenclature of personality disorders is a major error underpinned by political considerations rather than scientific considerations (Millon & Davies, 1996). Many diagnostic categories can be misused in forensic settings, yet this is not a good reason to obscure their existence and inhibit their study. It is the responsibility of the legal system to determine the influence that expert testimony has on issues including responsibility and risk; it is not the responsibility of those endeavoring to describe, measure and understand the disorder.

10. SEXUAL SADISM

Unlike Sadistic Personality Disorder, Sexual Sadism, remains an official diagnosis under DSM-IV (American Psychiatric Association, 1994). The primary feature of this disorder is that the individual experiences intense sexual arousal as a consequence of fantasies, sexual urges or behaviors that entail real – not simulated – acts during which their victim is subjected to physical and psychological suffering. It is the suffering of the victim that leads to sexual arousal. For example, one of Britain's most notorious serial killers, Ian Brady, recorded the screams of children he was strangling to death; he replayed these recordings before having sexual intercourse with his lover, Myra Hindley.

Sexual sadism tends to be a chronic disorder which onsets in adolescence or early adulthood. The range of behavior exhibit by sexual sadists is wide-ranging, and may include forcing –by verbal means– the victim to say words of particular significance to the perpetrator, or to carry out particular acts, but it may also include the use of physical methods – restraints, whipping, beating, burning, strangling, cutting, mutilation and torture– to terrify and subjugate the victim. In the extreme case, sexual sadism can lead to murder (Dietz, Hazelwood & Warren, 1990). Quinsey (1990) has described the wide-ranging nature of sexual sadistic behavior and emphasized that most individuals who met the diagnostic criteria for Sexual Sadism never physically damage another person: he suggests that the evidence available from pornographic literature and research on the sexual fantasies of 'normal men' implies that sexually sadistic thoughts and fantasies are not uncommon (Crepault & Couture, 1980; Deitz, Hazelwood & Warren, 1990).

Deviant sexual arousal and deviant sexual fantasies appear to underpin the development and maintenance of sexual sadism. In some early work using phallometric methods, Abel, Becker, Blanchard, and Djenderedjian (1977) found that sexual sadists exhibited disproportionately large penile changes in response to audio-taped descriptions of rapes as compared with non-sadistic rapists. (Brittain, 1970; MacCulloch, Snowden, Wood, & Mills, 1983; Prentky, Burgess, Rokous, Lee, Hartman, Ressler, & Douglas, 1989). Clinical case material has been used to identify the powerful interplay between deviant fantasy and deviant arousal. MacCulloch et al. (1983) argued that as fantasies develop, and of themselves no longer generate sufficient sexual arousal, the offender engages in behavioral 'try-outs' – for example, tracking a female down a dark street, or pretending to bump into a victim and thereby touching her private parts. Elements of the behavioral 'try-out' are then incorporated into fantasies which are used during masturbation: a downward cycle of progressively more serious offending develops. This is a powerful process. Prentky et al. (1989) argued that "Indeed, the selective reinforcement of deviant fantasies through paired association with masturbation over a protracted period may help to explain not only the power of fantasies but why they are so refractory to extinction." (p. 890).

Often by studying prototypical examples of a disorder we can grasp the essence of the disorder. Certain serial killers represent this prototype and by studying these cases the interplay between psychopathy, sadism and serial killing can be discerned. Dietz et al. (1990) provided a systematic account of cases from the most extreme end of the spectrum of sexual sadists, the sadistic murderer – "the sadist unencumbered by ethical, societal or legal inhibitions" (p. 163). They provided a quotation from a sadistic murderer which specifies the sine qua non of the disorder "Sadism: the wish to inflict pain on others is not that essence of sadism. One essential impulse: to have complete mastery over another person, to make him/her a helpless object of our will, to become the absolute ruler over her, to become her God, to do with her as one pleases. To humiliate her, to enslave her, are means to this end, and the most important radical aim is to make her suffer since there is no greater power over another person than that of inflicting pain on her to force her to undergo suffering without her being able to defend herself. The pleasure in the complete domination over another person is the very essence of the Sadistic drive" (p. 165).

Thus, many of their cohort of offenders used methods of torture and humiliation to instill morbid fear in their victims, they exercised the ultimate control – the power of life and death – over their victims by resuscitating their near-dead victims in order that they could subject them to further torture. Stone (1998) has described this as the Roman emperor syndrome: "The quest in the sadistic killer is for something even beyond omnipotent control: the quest is instead for the complete subjugation and the slow and painful destruction of other human beings" (p. 351).

The vast majority of the killers studied by Dietz et al. (1990) were known to be highly organized and to have planned their crimes carefully. They studied law enforcement techniques in order to minimizes the possibility of detection, they prepared their equipment – torture rooms, sound-proofed vans with disabled locks – they collected the tools and supplies necessary for the disposal of the bodies and they acquired the means for recording their victims suffering – tape recorders and video recorders – in order that they could relive the experiences, and sharpen their fantasies after the killing. They committed their crimes in a highly methodical manner, a manner characterized by the lack of any emotion; this contrasts markedly with the high emotion states that typify most violent offenses. Stone (1998) identified 5 steps that are common in the approaches used by sadistic killers in relation to their victims. First, they have the capability to identify vulnerable and passive female victims. In the second step, they use their superficial charm to win the affection of the victim by being apparently loving and considerate. On the third step, the victim is persuade to engage in a range of sexual practice including bondage, partaking in sexual videos and the use of dildoes. On the fourth step, the victim is progressively disengaged and isolated from her family and friends; jealousy and possessiveness being the mechanisms employed by the sadist to achieve the desired level of isolation. The victim may be further subjugated by being only provided with paltry sums for her needs. By the final step, the victim is powerless, and unable to resist the physical and psychological abuse meted out by her tormentor. Ultimately, as in the case of Ted Bundy, this may result in murder.

11. SEXUAL SADISM AND PSYCHOPATHY

Hart and Hare (1997) argued that there is likely to be an association between sexual sadism and psychopathy: among serial killers this certainly appears to be true (Stone, 1998). More generally, two studies of adult male offenders have found modest correlations between PCL-R scores and degree of sexual arousal to violent stimuli measured by phallometric assessment procedures ($r = .21$ in Quinsey, Rice, & Harris, 1995; $r = 0.28$ in Serin, Malcolm, Khanna, & Barbaree, 1994). More recently, Dempster and Hart (1996) found that among male juveniles charged with murder or attempted murder, those who were classified as sexual homicide perpetrators had significantly higher PCL-R scores than other types of offenders. The association between sexually deviant preferences and psychopathy may not be a simple relationship. Evidence from Rice and Harris (1997) suggests that there may be a synergistic relationship between these two characteristics and sexual recidivism. Psychopathic individuals who, on phallometric assessment, display strong preference for deviant stimuli –in particular stimuli concerned with sexual behavior with children– rape cues or violence cues of a non-sexual nature, had disproportionately higher rates of sexual recidivism than did other groups of offenders. Among adolescent sex offenders the combination of psychopathy and deviant sexual arousal is highly predictive of recidivism in general (Gretton, O'Shaughnessy, & Hare, 1998). These findings clearly have potential importance for risk assessments.

The nature and value of the construct of SPD remains elusive. The stage of development perhaps parallels the stage of development of the construct of psychopathy before the development of the PCL-R. If we are to develop an understanding of the complex interplay between psychopathy, sadism and serial killing, it is necessary to develop a more sophisticate understanding of SPD. It will be intriguing to discover whether the deletion of the SPD criteria from the DSM results in the extinction of the construct from clinical and research literatures (Widiger, 1995). If the construct is to develop it must encompass the affective and cognitive aspects of the disorder that have been identified as central within the clinical literature (Fiester & Gay, 1991, 1995; Millon & Davies, 1996). When sufficient data are available, the presence or other wise of a coherent latent trait needs to be determined using modern psychometric procedures (Embretson, 1996; Nunnally & Bernstein, 1994; Steinberg & Thissen, 1996). The relevance of particular items, and the amount of information they contribute to the construct, can be evaluated directly through the use of Item Response Theory methods (e.g., Cooke & Michie, 1997; King, King, Fairbank, Schlenger & Surface, 1993). It is only by developing more sophisticated measures of SPD, that we can begin to understand the complex interplay between SPD, psychopathy and serial killing.

REFERENCES

Abel, G. G.; Becker, J. V.; Blanchard, E. B. & Djenderedjian, A. (1977): "Differentiating sexual aggressives with penile measures", *Criminal Justice and Behavior*, 5, pp. 315-332.

American Psychiatric Association (1987): *Diagnostic and statistical manual of mental disorders* (3rd ed.), Washington DC, American Psychiatric Association.

Berger, P.: Unpublished raw data, quote in Fiester & Gay (1995).

Berger, P.; Berner, W.; Bolterauer, J.; Gutierrez, K. & Berger, K. (1999): "Sadistic personality disorder in sex offenders: relationship to antisocial personality disorder and sexual sadism", *Journal of Personality Disorders*, 13 (2), pp. 175-186.

Berner, W.; Berger, P.; Gutierrez, K.; Jordan, K. & Berger, K. (1992): "The role of personality disorder in the treatment of sex offenders", Journal of Offender Rehabilitation, 18, pp. 26-37.

Brittain, R. P. (1970): "The sadistic murderer", *Medicine, Science and the Law*, 10, pp. 198-207. Cleckley, H. (1976): *The mask of sanity* (5th ed.), St Louis, Mosby.

Crepault, C. & Couture, M. (1980): "Men's erotic fantasies", *Archives of Sexual Behavior*, 9, pp. 565-581. Cooke, D. J.; Forth, A. & Hare, R. D. (1998): *Psychopathy: theory, research and implications for society*, Kluwer Academic Publishers.

Cooke, D. J. & Michie, C. (1997): "An item response theory analysis of the Hare Psychopathy Checklist-Revised", *Psychological Assessment*, 9(1), pp. 3-14.

Cooke, D. J. & Michie, C. (1999a): *Refining the construct of psychopathy: Towards a hierarchical model* (unpub).

Cooke, D. J. & Michie, C. (1999b): "Psychopathy across cultures: North America and Scotland Compared", *Journal of Abnormal Psychology*, 108(1), pp. 55-68.

Cooke, D. J.; Michie, C.; Hart, S. D. & Hare, R. D. (1998): "The functioning of the Screening Version of the Psychopathy Checklist-Revised: An item response theory analysis", *Psychological Assessment*, 11 (1), pp. 3-13.

Cornell, D. G.; Warren, J.; Hawk, G.; Stafford, E.; Oram, G. & Pine, D.: "Psychopathy in Instrumental and Reactive Violent Offenders", *Journal of Consulting and Clinical*, 64 (4), pp. 783-790.

Dietz, P. E.; Hazelwood, R. R. & Warren, J. (1990): "The sexually sadistic criminal and his offenses", *Bulletin of the American Academy of Psychiatry and the Law*, 18(2), pp. 163-178.

Dempster, R. J. & Hart, S. D. (1996): *Utility of the FBI's crime classification manual; coverage, reliability, and validity for adolescent murders*, Hilton Head, South Carolina. Paper presented at the biennial meeting of the American Psychology-Law Society (APA Div. 41).

Embretson, S. E. (1996): "The new rules of measurement", *Psychological Assessment*, 8(4), pp. 341-349.

Fiester, S. J. & Gay, M. (1991): "Sadistic personality disorder: A review of data and recommendations for DSM-IV", *Journal of Personality Disorders*, 5(4), pp. 376-385.

Feister, S. & Gay, M. (1995): "Sadistic Personality Disorder", in W. J. Livesley (ed.), *The DSM-IV personality disorders*, New York, Guilford, pp. 329-340.

Freiman, K. & Widiger, T. A.: Unpublished data.

Fuller, A. K.; Blashfield, R. K.; Miller, M. & Hester, T. (1992): "Sadistic and self-defeating personality disorder criteria in a rural clinic sample", *Journal of Clinical Psychology*, 48(6), pp. 827-831.

Gay, M.: "Sadistic personality disorders among child abusers", in Anonymous, *Vol. Psychiatric diagnosis, victimization and women*, Symposium presented at the 142nd annual meeting of the American Psychiatric Association, San Francisco.

Hart, S. D. & Hare, R. D. (1995): "Commentary on antisocial personality disorder: the DSM-IV field trial", in W. J. Livesley (ed.), *The DSM-IV personality disorders*, New York, Guilford, pp. 127-134.

Hart, S. D. & Hare, R. D. (1997): "Psychopathy: Assessment and association with criminal conduct", in D. M. Stoff, J. Maser & J. Brieling (eds.), *Handbook of antisocial behavior*, New York, Wiley.

King, D. W.; King, L. A.; Fairbank, J. A.; Schlenger, W. E. & Surface, C. R. (1993): "Enhancing the precision of the Mississippi Scale for Combat-Related Posttraumatic Stress Disorder: an application of Item Response Theory", *Psychological Assessment*, 5, pp. 457-471.

Krafft-Ebing, R. (1898): *Psychopathia sexualis* (10th ed.), Stutgart, Enke.

Hare, R. D. (1970): *Psychopathy: theory and research*, New York, Wiley.

Hare, R. D. (1991), *Manual for the Revised Psychopathy Checklist*, (1st ed.), Toronto, Multi-Health Systems.

Hare, R. D. (1996): "Psychopathy: a clinical construct whose time has come", *Criminal Justice and Behavior*, 23, pp. 25-34.

Harpur, T. J.; Hakstian, A. & Hare, R. D. (1988): "Factor structure of the Psychopathy Checklist", *Journal of Consulting and Clinical Psychology*, 56, pp. 741-747.

Hart, S. D.; Dutton, D. G. & Newlove, T. (1993): "The prevalence of personality disorder among wife assaulters", *Journal of Personality Disorders*, 7(4), pp. 329-341.

Hart, S. D. & Hare, R. D. (1995): "Commentary on antisocial personality disorder: the DSM-IV field trial", in W. J. Livesley (ed.), *The DSM-IV personality disorders*, New York, Guilford, pp. 127-134.

Hartung, C. M. & Widiger, T. A. (in press): "Gender differences in the diagnosis of mental disorders: Conclusions and controversies of DSM-IV", *Psychological Bulletin*.

MacCulloch, M. J.; Snowden, P. R.; Wood, P. J. & Mills, H. E. (1983): "Sadistic fantasy, sadistic behavior and offending", *British Journal of Psychiatry*, 143, pp. 20-29.

Millon, T. (1981): *Disorders of personality*, New York, Wiley.

Millon, T. & Davis, R. D. (1996): *Disorders of personality DSM-IV and beyond* (2nd ed.), New York, Wiley.

Millon, T. & Tringone, R.: unpublished raw data, quote in Fiester & Gay (1995).

Nunnally, J.C. & Bernstein, I. H. (1994): "*Psychometric theory*" (3rd ed.), McGraw-Hill Inc.

Prentky, R.; Burgess, A. W.; Rokous, F.; Lee, A.; Hartman, C.; Ressler, R. & Douglas, J. (1989): "The presumptive role of fantasy in serial sexual homicide", *American Journal of Psychiatry*, 146 (7), pp. 887-891.

Quinsey, V. L. (1990): "Sexual violence", in P. Bowden & R. Bluglass (eds.), *Principles and practice of forensic psychiatry*, Edinburgh, Churchill Livingstone, pp. 563-570.

Quinsey, V. L.; Rice, M. E. & Harris, G. T. (1995): "Actuarial prediction of sexual recidivism", *Journal of Interpersonal Violence*, 10, pp. 85-105.

Raine, A. (1993): *The psychopathology of crime: Criminal behavior as a clinical disorder*, San Diego, Academic Press.

Rice, M. E. & Harris, G. T. (1997): "Cross-validation and extension of the Violence Risk Appraisal Guide for child molesters and rapists", *Law and Human Behavior*, 21 (2), pp. 231-241.

Serin, R. C.; Malcolm, P. B.; Khanna, A. & Barbaree, H. E. (1994): "Psychopathy and deviant sexual arousal in incarcerated sexual offenders", *Journal of Interpersonal Violence*, 9, pp. 3-11.

Spitzer, R. L.; Fiester, S. J.; Gay, M. & Pfohl, B. (1991): "Is sadistic personality disorder a valid diagnosis? The results of a survey of forensic psychiatrists", *American Journal of Psychiatry*, 148 , pp. 875-879.

Steinberg, L. & Thissen, D. (1996): "Uses of Item Response Theory and the testlet concept in the measurement of psychopathology", *Psychological Measurement*, 1(1), pp. 81-97.

Stone, M. (1998): "Sadistic personality in murderers", in T. Millon, E. Simonsen, M. Birket-Smith & R. D. Davies (eds.), *Psychopathy: Antisocial, criminal and violent behavior*, London, Guilford, pp. 346-355.

Storr, A. (1990): "Sadomasochism", in P. Bowden & R. Bluglass (eds.), *Principles and practice of forensic psychiatry*, Edinburgh, Churchill Livingstone, pp. 711-716.

Widiger, T. A. (1995): "Deletion of Self-Defeating and Sadistic Personality Disorders", in W. J. Livesley (ed.), *The DSM-IV personality disorders*, New York, Guilford, pp. 359-373.

Widiger, T. A.; Frances, R. J.; Spitzer, R. L. & Williams, J. B. W. (1988): "The DSM-IIIR personality disorders: An overview", *American Journal of Psychiatry*, 145, pp. 786-795.

Widiger, T. A. & Trull, T. J. (1994): "Personality disorders and violence", in J. Monahan & J. S. Henry Steadman (eds.), *Violence and mental disorder: Developments in risk assessment*, Chicago IL, University of Chicago Press.

PART III

PSYCHOSOCIAL ASPECTS AND TREATMENT

Chapter 8

PSYCHOSOCIAL CONTRIBUTIONS TO PSYCHOPATHY AND VIOLENCE[1]

Joan McCord
Department of Criminal Justice, Temple University, Philadelphia, Pennsylvania, USA

1. INTRODUCTION

Many, perhaps most, psychopaths are sometimes violent. Psychopaths also count heavily among criminally violent populations (Hare & McPherson, 1984). Because of this strong overlap between psychopathy and violent criminals, research regarding the contributions that psychological and social conditions make to the one are confounded by their contributions to the other. Nevertheless, it is well to attempt identification of the psychopaths among those who are violent. Failure to make such identification confounds disease with its symptoms. Imagine, as a parallel, attempting to find the causes and cures for fevers without looking for underlying differentiation based on clusters of concomitant symptoms. One ought not expect the same correlates or causes for violence among psychopaths and violence among others. Nor is it likely that the means for preventing violence will be the same for people motivated in different ways. Therefore, the identification of psychopaths among those who are violent is likely to contribute to a clearer understanding of the causes of violence and to its control.

Several recent studies have indicated that identification of psychopathy as a particular disorder may be useful for the prevention of violence. For example, Lynam (1996), noting the similarity of children who display both conduct disorder and hyperactivity to a description of psychopaths, also pointed out that these children are likely to begin their antisocial activities at younger ages, to be more actively antisocial, and to commit more severe

[1] The author thanks her hosts of the Queen Sofia Center for the Study of Violence for a fascinating conference where an earlier version of this paper was presented and Adrian Raine for helpful comments on that version.

crimes than those children who were diagnosed with conduct disorder or hyperactivity, but not both. As part of a birth-cohort study in Dunedin, New Zealand, Caspi and Silva (1995) identified five "temperamental groups" of children on the basis of ratings for lack of control, eagerness to explore new situations, and withdrawal or sluggishness at the age of 3 years. One group of children, considered to be "undercontrolled," had scored high on irritability and distractivility; they had difficulty in sustaining attention and seemed emotionally labile. When they were 18, the subjects responded to questions describing their own personalities. The authors characterize the behavior at the age of 18 for the children who had been undercontrolled at the age of 3 as "high on a constellation of traits that index low behavioral constraint; they described themselves as danger-seeking and impulsive... they said they were prone to respond with strong negative emotions to everyday events" (p. 495). The characteristics describing 18-year olds are remarkably similar to those that have characterized psychopathic personalities. Lynam (1997) suggests that "classification schemes proposed for conduct disorders have not provided predictive validity primarily because of an overreliance on behavioral descriptors (e.g., the type, pattern, developmental sequence, or timing of conduct problems)" (p. 425).

The usefulness of a psychopathic diagnosis has been tested also in a study of adult males released from a maximum security psychiatric hospital after a minimum stay of two years of treatment in a therapeutic community program (Harris, Rice, & Cormier, 1991). The released men had been classified as psychopaths (N=52) or non-psychopaths (N=114), on the basis of Hare's Psychopathy Checklist and prison files. Researchers did not know the follow-up information indicating which of the men were violent recidivists. Among the non-psychopaths, 21% committed a violent crime; among the psychopaths, 77% had done so. For every age, including those over 40 at the time of their release, a higher proportion of the psychopaths were violent recidivists. The Psychopathy Checklist scores provided a more effective basis for predicting violent recidivism than did criminal histories. Furthermore, when entered into a regression with prior criminal histories already entered, scores on the Psychopathy Checklist raised R from .312 to .447, a highly significant increase. By way of contrast, Harris and his co-authors noted that predictions based on diagnosis for antisocial personality disorder did not perform as well.

It seems safe to say that psychopaths constitute a small proportion of criminals apprehended for violent offenses. The evidence for this claim is that among violent criminals, only a handful (estimated in one study as 4.8% of all juveniles referred to court for a violent offense) have been convicted for more than three violent offenses (Snyder, 1998). Nevertheless, the small number of criminals who are psychopaths contribute disproportionately to the amount of crime so disturbing to civilized communities.

2. CHARACTERIZING PSYCHOPATHS

Of course there are many meaningful ways to subtype violent offenders. The dichotomy produced by differentiating psychopaths from non-psychopaths should be taken only as a step toward understanding a group of people who share a class of characteristics that make them particularly dangerous.

A variety of attempts have been made to develop useful subtypes among Psychopaths. For example, Ben Karpman (1941) distinguished between the "idiopathic" psychopath and the "symptomatic" psychopath. Blackburn (1975) identified four types, all of whom had high scores on the Pd scale of the Minnesota Multiphasic Personality Inventory (MMPI). Others have identified sexual psychopaths, aggressive psychopaths, and affectionless psychopaths to reflect characteristics thought to be particularly salient regarding the puzzling individuals who seem not to fear what others fear and to ignore common strictures against misbehavior. Although neither a single definition, nor particular criterial characteristics have been universally established, Hare and Cox (1978) showed that identification of psychopaths can be carried out reliably.

Psychopaths have long been recognized to be among the most dangerous people, whether inside or outside of prison. They are dangerous in part because they have a high threshold for physical pain. This feature of psychopaths has been demonstrated in several ways. Schmauk (1970) gave painful shocks to imprisoned primary psychopaths, imprisoned neurotic psychopaths, farm workers, and attendants at a state hospital. Alternative "punishments" included loosing money or gaining disapproval for wrong responses. A maze was used to measure effects of various punishments on learning. The psychopaths learned the maze as well as the non-criminals did when the lessons came with monetary or social indications of wrong choices. They were less responsive, however, to the shocks. Because they learned when their anxiety increased, Schmauk concluded that primary psychopaths have fewer stimuli that arouse their anxiety.

Physical threat generally fails to inhibit psychopaths although their actions appear to be guided exclusively by their perceptions of self-interest. Nevertheless, in at least one study of convicts (Berg, 1974), those classified as sociopaths (psychopaths) described themselves as warm-hearted and unselfish as well as daring and adventurous. Because they are "daring," as Gatzke and Raine (2000) noted, "the reliance on punishment as a deterrent is least likely to work in the very group that will most likely be committing the most crimes" (p. 53).

Among violent criminals, psychopaths are likely to be differentiated by being younger at first arrest. Because psychopaths have little empathy or attachment to people, they are likely to do things that injure others without regard to how their misbehavior might make their parents or other caregivers feel. Psychopaths are also likely to be identifiable by the high frequency of their offending. Because psychopaths are impulsive, when something angers them, they are likely to react aggressively. If they see something they want, they are likely to take it. High rates of recidivism reflect the characteristic impulsiveness of psychopaths (Kosson, Smith, & Newman, 1990).

3. PSYCHOPATHY IN HISTORICAL PERSPECTIVE

Philippe Pinel apparently originated the clinical concept of psychopathy in 1801, when he coined the term *manie sans délire* as a diagnosis for people who exhibited uncontrolled rage coupled with normal intellectual functioning. James Prichard interjected the concept into British criminology through his *Treatise on Insanity and Other Disorders Affecting the Mind*, published in 1837. Prichard referred to mania without mental defects as "moral insanity," an insanity of judgment rather than of intelligence.

In an argument that strikes a modern chord, B. A. Morel (1857), one of the most influential early criminal anthropologists pointed out that heredity involves transmission from parents to children of organic dispositions, rather than specific mental or physical symptoms. It remained for Cesare Lombroso to place psychopathy at the center of criminological theory. His book, L'uomo delinquente, published in 1876, provided a summary of the then-popular theories regarding crime as a manifestation of degeneracy. He added physical measurements to distinguish among crime-typed individuals. Ascribing moral insanity to the "born criminal," Lombroso believed the disease was a variant of epilepsy. Gina Lombroso-Ferrero (1911) described her father as the first to recognize the importance of "irresistible atavistic impulse" to explain the crimes of those whom others had diagnosed as morally insane. "They differed from ordinary people," she wrote of psychopaths, "because they hated the very persons who to normal beings are the nearest and dearest, parents, husbands, wives, and children, and because their inhuman deeds seemed to cause them no remorse" (p. 52).

Havelock Ellis (1890) championed the work of the criminal anthropologists from the continent to his English-speaking audience. Ellis urged, however, use of the term "instinctive" rather than "born" or "congenital" because of difficulty in determining the role of biology in formation of moral insanity. "The instinctive criminal, in his fully developed form, is a moral monster. In him the absence of guiding or inhibiting social instincts is accompanied by unusual development of the sensual and self-seeking impulses," (p. 2) he wrote.

From the mid-nineteenth to the mid-twentieth century, many scientists viewed psychopathy as heritable degeneracy. Famously, Dugdale (1877) published the results of tracing the "Jukes" family. The relevant family origin, Dugdale reported, began in "one of the crime cradles of the State of New York" (p. 13) around 1792. Dugdale traced the genealogy of the Jukes through seven generations. Among the conclusions he reached was that "Environment tends to produce habits which may become hereditary, especially so in pauperism and licentiousness, if it should be sufficiently constant to produce modifications of cerebral tissue" (p. 66). Under the auspices of the Carnegie Institution, a leading research center for the Eugenics Movement, Estabrook (1916) traced 2820 relatives in the Jukes family to 1915. Estabrook concluded that degeneracy, not criminality`, was inherited.

Enrico Ferri (1897), often considered to be one of the founding fathers of modern criminology, carefully distinguishing between the "congenital, incorrigible, and habitual criminals" and the occasional criminal who was not to be seen as having inherited disabilities. He argued that moral insensibility served to identify habitual criminals. Ferri concluded that punishment was ineffective: "Punishment, in fact, by its special effect as a legal deterrent, acting as a psychological motive, will clearly be unable to neutralize the constant and hereditary action of climate, customs, increase of population, agricultural production, economic and political crises, which statistics invariably exhibit as the most potent factors of the growth or diminution of criminality" (p. 92).

This was a period during which the eugenics movement was building momentum. Around 1900, according to Haller's history of the Eugenics movement (1963/1984), Mendel's 1865 paper demonstrating the statistical probabilities of inheritance in peas had resurfaced and the laws of heredity had been independently rediscovered by three investigators. These coincidental events contributed significantly to the push to control what were viewed to be inherited depravities.

Between 1899 and 1907, Dr. Harry C. Sharp, a surgeon for the Indiana reformatory, performed 465 vasectomies on inmates (Fink, 1938). In 1907, Indiana passed a law using vasectomy as punishment for criminals, idiots, rapists, and imbeciles. By 1915, 13 states had laws authorizing sterilization. Partly because of testing brought about by World War I, assumptions about the link between feeblemindedness and crime were brought into question. Army testing and the aftermath of developments in the fields of psychology and psychiatry broadened the range of influences thought to lead to habitual criminality.

4. THE DEVELOPMENT OF PSYCHOPATHY

Even in childhood, psychopaths are impulsive, aggressive, emotionally isolated people whose craving for excitement is curbed neither by social norms nor by conscience (Bender, 1947; Cleckley, 1941/1976; Hare & Cox,

1978; Klinteberg, Humble, & Schalling, 1992; McCord, 1983; McCord & McCord, 1964; Schulsinger, 1977; Siddle, 1977). Describing such children, as they appeared in records of a psychiatric clinic, Lee Robins (1966) wrote: "Such boys had a history of truancy, theft, staying out late, and refusing to obey parents. They lied gratuitously, and showed little guilt over their behavior. They were generally irresponsible about being where they were supposed to be or taking care of money. They were interested in sexual activities and had experimented with homosexual relationships. Their parents complained of their bed wetting and poor grooming" (p. 157). It is easy to understand, therefore, why many have assumed that psychopathy is congenital.

Although "psychopathy" refers to a type of personality, a type that some have argued has biological roots, there are grounds for believing that social interaction markedly contributed to the personality of psychopaths. Indeed, recognition of a social contribution to the personality of psychopaths has led some researchers to call these people "sociopaths" (e.g., Allen, Dinitz, Foster, Goldman, & Lindner, 1976; Beran & Allen, 1981; Berg, 1974; Cloninger, Reich, & Guze, 1975; Lykken, 1957; Robins, 1966; Schmauk, 1970; Schuckit, 1973; Wolman, 1987.)

Many studies of children whose behavior brought them to the attention of authorities also revealed backgrounds of parental rejection. In one early study, a psychotherapist in a reform school found that all of his psychopathic delinquents had been rejected by their parents as young children (Partridge, 1928). In another study, 23 of 25 children in a State Psychiatric Institute were found to have had rejecting mothers (Field, 1940). Probably the most definitive work of this genre came from the studies by Lauretta Bender. As a clinician at New York's Bellevue Hospital, Bender examined hundreds of child psychopaths. She found that all the psychopathic children had experienced emotional deprivation, neglect, or discontinuous affectional relationships.

Studies based on examining consequences of rejection, rather than backgrounds of psychopaths, confirmed a link between aggression and emotional isolation. William Newell (1934, 1936) examined 75 rejected children from Cleveland Public Schools and compared them with 82 pupils in a third or fifth grade classroom in Baltimore. He found that the rejected children were much more likely to be aggressive. David Levy (1937) studied rejected children undergoing treatment at the Institute for Child Guidance in New York. He learned that the children lacked emotional depth, had difficulties learning from experience, and were extremely aggressive. Percival Symonds (1939) used a matched design to compare 31 pairs of children, one of whom in each pair was rejected and the other accepted by their parents. The children were matched for age, sex, grade in school, social background, and intelligence. Based on the mothers' reports of their behavior, Symonds concluded that the rejection resulted in children becoming restless, emotionally unstable, apathetic, and generally antagonistic toward society and its institutions.

In his careful and influential analysis of the important role played by maternal care for the healthy development of children, John Bowlby (1951) identified three types of maternal deprivation as contributing to affectionless psychopathy. These involve a lack of opportunity for forming attachments to a mother figure, temporary deprivation of contact with the mother figure for a period of months during the child's first four years, and repeated shifts in caretakers during early childhood. Bowlby pointed out that affectionless psychopathic children grow up to become affectionless psychopathic parents who rear psychopathic children. Bowlby decried the emphasis placed on heritability because he saw maternal behavior as accounting for the generational transmission of psychopathy.

Robins (1966), however, reported no clear relationship between parental rejection and psychopathy among the clinic children she had retraced as adults. In fact, even the relation between parental repudiation, defined in terms of initiating action to remove a child from the home, and psychopathy disappeared when the behavior of the child and the parents was taken into account. In a work aimed at critically assessing contributions of maternal deprivation to developmental problems, Rutter (1972) suggested that focus had wrongly been placed on mothers. "In the writer's view," he wrote, "theories of mothering have frequently been too mechanical in equating separation with bond disruption, too restricted in regarding the mother as the only person important in a child's life, and too narrow in considering love as the only important element in maternal care" (p. 51). Reflecting on the relationship between parental rejection and psychopathy, Herbert Quay (1977) suggested that the noxious behavior of their infants, especially in relation to an abnormal desire for stimulation, leads to the types of punishment and rejection others claimed caused the child's behavior.

Characteristics that identify psychopaths -- impulsivity, aggressiveness, lack of close ties, desire for excitement, absence of remorse for transgressions, and frequent norm violations -- can be traced to several social sources. Such tracing ought not, however, be taken to suggest that there are no biological contributions to their origins. Rather, interactions between biological and experiential events are so central to development that their separation would properly be characterized as one of focus.

5. SOCIAL INFLUENCES AND NEUROBIOCHEMICAL CORRELATES

Undoubtedly, some differences in personality (which are sometimes considered to be temperament) have biological roots. Which roots are biological in origin is, however, less than clear. In this section, I discuss some of the biological evidence and grounds for believing that biological differences may reflect earlier social experiences.

Perinatal complications have been linked with aggressive antisocial behavior. For example, Kandel and Mednick (1991) found that such complications predicted violent criminality in a Danish sample. Brennan, Mednick, and Raine (1997) found that perinatal complications, especially with low SES, predicted disinhibitions at the age of 11 in a Mauritius sample. Yet among low-birthweight, premature infants, home visits have been shown to improve cognitive scores and behavior for as long as 36 months (Brooks-Gunn et al. 1993) and to reduce criminal behavior for many years (Olds, et al., 1998). These studies provide grounds for believing that adverse effects from perinatal complications may be attributed to a deficient environment as much as to the initial trauma.

Adrian Raine (1996) reviewed evidence regarding autonomic nervous system factors related to the types of behavior for which psychopaths are noted. In terms of arousal, Raine (1996a) concluded that studies of resting heart rate yielded "striking support for under-arousal in antisocial and aggressive children" (p. 47). Elsewhere, Raine (1996b) suggested that low heart rate "may predispose to the development of fearlessness, which predisposes to violent and antisocial behavior" (p.164).

Biochemical studies have implicated serotonergic functioning in relation to aggression. Knoblich and King (1992) suggested that because 5-HT becomes active when conflicting stimuli are present, low levels of serotonin may result in disinhibition, though not in initial arousal of aggressive responses. Coccaro (1995) showed strong negative correlations between cerebrospinal fluid levels of 5-HIAA and aggression. He also reported a double-blind, placebo-controlled study in which male prison inmates received lithium, a drug known to increase serotonin brain activity, on some trials. The study yielded striking results: "Impulsive-aggressive actions of subjects treated with lithium, as routinely recorded by correctional personnel, were reduced to near zero by the end of the third month. Subjects treated with placebo showed no reduction in these behaviors. Moreover, lithium-treated subjects who were crossed-over to placebo in a double-blind fashion lost the gains they made during the trial within a month off active lithium treatment" (p. 41). In another study that measured blood serotonin, in a 21-year-old general population, Moffitt et al. (1997) found that high blood serotonin reflected violence among males, whether violence was measured in self-reports or by official criminal records. Violence was particularly likely when high blood serotonin boys had been reared in families that exposed them to conflict. Goyer and Semple (1996) used PET scan data to link serotonin receptors in the frontal cortex to patients' aggressive behavior.

The density of platelet membrane receptors for 5-HT have been found to be inversely related to frequent parental physical punishment and anger (Pine et al., 1996). And in a fenfluramine challenge study of boys, serotonergic activity and aggression has been shown to be influenced by poor social environments (Pine et al., 1997).

Neuropsychological tests have identified problems in language skills and self control attributed to executive functions of the brain. As Moffitt (1997) noted in a comprehensive review of neuropsychology and antisocial behavior, test scores have identified such problems among subject who have abnormal electroencephalographic recordings from electrode sites in the front of the brain and show poor blood flow to the frontal lobes when measured in PET scans. The deficits, Moffitt suggests, manifest themselves in low verbal intelligence which can lead to a series of difficulties as infants mature.

Lower 5-HT (serotonin) function has been found among aggressive boys with aggressive parents than among aggressive boys without aggressive parents (Halperin, et al., 1997). This finding might be an indication of an inherited characteristic. On the other hand, if the aggressive parents create stress in the family, or if the mothers in such families smoke when pregnant, the link could be a result of environmental stress. A variety of studies indicate that the hypothalamic-pituitary-adrenal axis can be affected by prepartum environments as well as perinatal stress (King, 1996).

Gunnar and Barr (1998) report research that demonstrates how changes due to early experiences alter the brain's stress circuits affecting learning and physiological responses to stress and challenge. The authors note that until recently, "brain development was believed to be under strong genetic control" (p. 2). Yet recent research has shown the degree to which brain development is responsive to experiences. The authors conclude, "The cost of adapting to stressful life circumstances often results in loss of dendrites, synapses, and nerve cells" (p. 2). The article summarizes animal research that shows that early experiences govern how well the brain controls the magnitude and duration of glucocorticoid elevations. Such elevations are activated under stressful conditions and are likely to influence harmful effects of those stressful conditions. Increasing levels of glucocorticoids, the authors report, interfere with the ability to sustain attention and to focus on information. Experimental studies with monkeys and rats have shown that enhanced maternal care increases glucocorticoid receptors in the brain, resulting in reduced fear and decreased catecholamine responses to stressors. Another experiment with rhesus monkeys raised in peer groups without their mothers allowed some of the infant monkeys to control the timing of food, drinks, and treats. Another group of monkeys, yoked to the first, had no control over their own food, drinks, and treats, though they received these items whenever their partners requested them. The former group, those who could control their environments, were less fearful, more willing to explore, and when they matured, showed smaller HPA axis stress responses to anxiety-producing drugs. Another study reported by Gunnar and Barr (1998) showed that circumcised infants increased their cortisol production for about two hours after the operation. As compared with uncircumcised infants, the circumcised infants showed greater pain in stressful conditions as much as six months later.

Other types of research, using animal models, have shown that environmental enrichment increases synaptic connections in rats, and that restrictions on sight alter synaptic connections in cats (Greenough, Black, & Wallace, 1987). In a series of experiments on non-human animals, scientists have demonstrated that effects of various brain manipulations depend on experiences as well as surrounding chemistry (See Karli, 1996, for a review). For example, a rat's mouse-killing behavior in response to brain manipulations depended on whether or not it had prior experience with mice. A rat's opiate systems could be altered by maternal stress during the fetal period or by repeated separation from its mother shortly after birth. Thus, it seems clear that physiological events thought to be causally related to psychopathy depend essentially on experiences.

6. FAMILY SOCIALIZATION AND CHILD DEVELOPMENT

Crime, it should be noted, requires intentional action. Therefore, whether the contributing causes are biological or social, they must tap into the conscious mind of those who act intentionally. Both social and biological factors contribute to psychopathy, I suggest, by affecting the ways that individuals perceive their choices about behavior.

The focus of this section will be on socialization practices that seem to be related to incipient psychopathy. The section begins with infancy, taking a look at the types of socialization necessary to teach infants to accept and internalize social norms as well as whether to care about the ways others feel.

Several bits of evidence suggest that the impact of social conditions on personality may be considerable. For example, Riese (1990) compared 47 pairs of monozygotic, 39 pairs of same-sex dizygotic, and 72 pairs of opposite-sex dizygotic twins. Comparisons included tests for irritability, resistance to soothing, activity level when awake, activity level when asleep, reactivity to a cold disk on the thigh and to a pin prick, and responses to cuddling. Riese found significant correlations for both same-sex and opposite-sex dizygotic twins. Correlations among the monozygotic pairs were not significantly greater than those among dizygotic pairs. Riese concluded that "environment appears to account for most of the known variance for the neonatal temperament variables" (p. 1236).

Further evidence of the impact that social environments can have on what appears to be innate personality comes as a byproduct of a study of female neonates. The experiment began when the infants were 12 hours old and lasted 48 hours. Researchers randomly assigned 18 first-born healthy neonates to one of three conditions. Two of them involved using a recording of a mother saying such things as "Hi, baby, hello there." For these two conditions, the recording was played when an infant was alert, perhaps fussy or crying, between feedings. In one of the conditions, after the baby had heard the recording for five seconds, she was picked up and held to the experimenter's shoulder for 33 seconds before being replaced into the crib. In the second condition, the infant heard the recording as in the first, but was not lifted to the shoulder. The third condition was a control group in which the neonates were neither held nor exposed to the recording of a mother's voice during the first 60 hours of their lives. As anticipated, the randomly selected babies who were held were the ones who subsequently spent more time with their eyes open. Unexpectedly, after the experiment ended, they also spent more time crying. The authors concluded: "Because these infants had received many associations of the auditory stimulation and being picked up when they cried during the 48-hour training period, it is likely that they came to associate crying with being picked up" (Thoman, Korner, & Benson-Williams, 1977, p. 568). In short, the babies seem to have been taught to want to be held and to cry in order to communicate this.

Other evidence of learning among neonates comes from a study of infants shortly after their births. Each received a simple physical examinations at discharge from the hospital and again 24 hours later. The initial examinations resulted in sharp increases in cortisol, a sign of stress. Yet when the examination was repeated the next day, there was no cortisol increase among the newborn infants. The infants had apparently learned not to fear the examination (Gunnar, Connors, & Isensee, 1989). A second study provided evidence that the change in stress response to nonintrusive physical examinations cannot be attributed to age or repetition alone. The second study showed that learning effects were not found with pin pricks of the heel. Sharp increases in cortisol occurred after both the first and the second examinations involving heel pin pricks (Gunnar, Hertsgaard, Larson, & Rigatuso, 1992).

In normal households, newborn babies are cared for by adults who are responsive to their cries or movements indicative of hunger or other sources of pain or desire. Such responsiveness teaches infants that their discomfort can be alleviated by the actions of others. Very early, infants learn to recognize the smells and sounds of caregivers who attend them, with neonates showing a preference for their own mother's voice (DeCasper & Fifer, 1980; Schaal, 1988; Spence & DeCasper, 1987).

In some homes, however, no one responds to a baby's signs of need. Some of these homes are so neglecting of infants that even their physical well-being is jeopardized. In other homes, although the infant is fed enough to survive, it does not learn how to control an environment in order to obtain even essential sustenance. Absence of control, even without deprivation, appears to increase stress.

Stress-reducing effects of control occur even in very young children. For example, a study of one-year-old infants who had been frightened by a noisy toy showed that the infants found the same toy amusing when they could make the toy noisy themselves (Gunnar-Vongnechten, 1978).

Neglect is known to be an important risk factor for psychopathy (Bender, 1947; Hare, 1970; McCord & McCord, 1964; see also Hawkins, Herrenkohl, Farrington, Brewer, Catalano, & Harachi, 1998). The mechanisms linking neglect to violence appear to be partly through stress responses and their effects.

Animal models have shown that early stress increases the magnitude and duration of glucocorticoid responses. These glucocorticoid responses influence levels of cortisol on an amygdala corticotropin-releasing hormone which, in turn, can shrink dendrites and lead to cell death (Gunnar & Barr, 1998). At least in animal models, the process from stress through shrinking of dendrites and cell death seems to reduce attention span and self-control. Gunnar and Barr (1998) summarize this line of research by noting: "Frequent and prolonged exposure to elevated cortisol may affect the development of brain areas involved in memory, negative emotions, and attention regulation....Sensitive and responsive caregivers and secure emotional relationships in infancy and early childhood may protect the developing brain and reduce later stress reactivity" (p. 10).

Short attention span and hyperactivity as well as lack of self-control, or impulsiveness, are characteristics that have repeatedly been shown to be typical of psychopaths (Blackburn, 1975; Emmons & Webb, 1974; Hare, 1978; Harper, Morris, & Bleyerveld, 1972; McCord & McCord, 1964; Zuckerman, 1978). They are also predictive of violence (Farrington, 1989; Magnusson, Klinteberg, & Stattin, 1992; Mannuzza, Klein, Konig, & Giampino, 1989). Extrapolating from the studies of animal models the data suggest that impulsiveness and short attention spans may be responses to early deficits in an infant's control over the environment.

As mentioned above, psychopaths exhibit poor executive function and deficits in language. These defects, too, may be consequences of inadequate adult attention during infancy. Shortly after birth, infants begin to learn the language of those surrounding them. When infants are about a month old, they recognize significant cues from their environments (Camras, Malatesta,

& Izard, 1991). At 15 months, infants search for objects when an adult provides a novel name and by 16 months, infants seem capable of distinguishing between names for objects and idle use of sounds (Markman, 1994). Baldwin (1991) showed that infants identified cues from a speaker's eyes. Babies who were 16 months old learned a label when the speaker was looking at the same target as the baby, but if the speaker's attention was directed away from the object that attracted the baby's attention, the baby did not assign the label to the object (Baldwin, 1991). Neglected babies are unlikely to have the relevant adult interactions that would promote early acquisition of language.

We know that persistent criminals and psychopaths are relatively unresponsive to physical pains (Farrington, 1988; Hare, 1978; Hinton, O'Neill, M., Hamilton, S., & Burke, 1980; Lykken, 1957; Mednick, 1977; Rotenberg, 1978; Satterfield, 1987; Schalling, 1978; Schmauk, 1970; Siddle, 1977; Siegel, 1978; Spielberger, Kling, & O'Hagan, 1978; Wadsworth, 1976). Some theorize that this lack of responsiveness results in slow learning regarding what behavior is undesirable.

Compared with nonpsychopaths, psychopaths are less likely to exhibit fear in response to stimuli that provoke anxiety in normal people. David Lykken (1957), for example, compared the avoidance learning of imprisoned psychopaths with that of students, some of whom were in high school and some in a university. He found that the psychopaths were more likely to choose alternatives that resulted in their receiving shocks. Robert Hare (1978) compared psychopathic prisoners with nonpsychopathic inmates in terms of their responsiveness to loud (120 db) tones. The psychopaths showed smaller skin conductance responses. Hare linked the low levels of arousal to a reduction in inhibition and a lack of interest in the tasks that seem to arouse nonpsychopaths.

Studies of institutionalized infants indicate the degree to which caring about pains is a function of experience. Goldfarb (1945, 1958) reported his observations of institutionalized children who received little attention. One child sat on a radiator too hot for the teacher to touch. Another was observed cutting the palm of his own hand with sharp scissors. Another closed a door on her hand, injuring her finger so severely that it turned blue; but she did not cry or otherwise show pain. Another had a steel splinter removed from her cornea, where it had been imbedded for two days without any report of the injury. All the children gave pain responses to pin pricks, so that it was clear they had normal pain receptors. It seems fair to conclude that in an unresponsive environment, these children had learned to ignore their own injuries.

There is little reason to believe children who learn not to attend their own pains would notice the injuries of others. This lack of empathy is one of the characteristics noticed in psychopaths (Gough, 1948; Hare, 1990; McCord & McCord, 1964; Rotenberg, 1978).

During the first few months of life, normal children have learned to cry in response to the cry of another human being (Sagi & Hoffman, 1976; Simner, 1971). They have learned also to display emotions, with facial expressions akin to those found in adults. For example, by the third week infants sometimes smile with open eyes and contraction of the muscles circling the eyes. This early responsiveness may well be dependent upon interactions found in normally responsive families. When children are about a month old, pleasant sounds and soft touches produce smiles (Camras, Malatesta, & Izard, 1991).

In the absence of appropriate stimuli, infants are unlikely to smile. That is, they will not show the types of responses that subsequently tend to produce favorable reactions of others. Neglecting and abusing parents fail to provide environments conducive to learning how to smile. They therefore are likely to have children who do not behave in ways that elicit approval from others.

To some extent, children learn about how others feel by having those feelings expressed both physically, through gestures, and verbally. Abusing as well as neglecting parents spend little time communicating with their children (Kavanagh, Youngblade, Reid, & Fagot, 1988). The children are likely, therefore, to have little understanding of the thoughts or feelings of others (Perry & Perry, 1974).

Parental rejection and neglect are related not only to stress, relative immunity from pain, and lack of empathy, but also to high levels of aggression in children (Bowlby, 1940, 1951; Dornbusch, Carlsmith, Bushwall, Ritter, Leiderman, Hastorf, & Gross, 1985; Eron, Huesmann, & Zelli, 1991; Farrington, Gundry, & West, 1975; Goldfarb, 1945; Hirschi, 1969; Laub & Sampson, 1988; Liska & Reed, 1985; Loeber & Stouthamer-Loeber, 1986; McCord, 1983; Newell, 1934, 1936; Olweus, 1980; Wells & Rankin, 1988). Some (e.g., Hirschi, 1969) attribute the link between parental rejection or neglect and aggression to failures in attachment. They have argued that children must be willing to give up satisfactions gained through aggression in exchange for benefits gained from being a part of a social unit.

7. PERPETUATION OF AGGRESSION AND EFFECTS OF PUNISHMENT

At least under some conditions, childhood aggression tends to be perpetuated (Cairns, Cairns, Neckerman, Ferguson, & Gariépy, 1989; Farrington, 1992; McCord & Ensminger, 1997; Olweus, 1979). Aggression is particularly likely to continue if it is not coupled with prosocial behavior (Pulkkinen & Tremblay, 1992; Tremblay, 1991). Aggressive, uncontrolled behavior during childhood serves as a specific predictor for crimes against persons (McCord & Ensminger, 1997; Stattin & Magnusson, 1989).

Several studies have linked aggressive or violent criminal behavior to earlier exposure to harsh physical punishments (e.g., Egeland & Sroufe, 1981; Farrington, 1978; Herrenkohl & Herrenkohl, 1981; Main & Goldwyn, 1984; McCord, 1983; Weiss, Dodge, Bates, & Pettit, 1992; Widom, 1989). In one longitudinal study, effects of physical punishments were studied after checking that their use was not predicted from prior misbehavior of the child (McCord, 1997a). In this study, parental warmth and punitiveness were measured from case records that included direct observations for an average of five and one-half years of visits to the homes of more than two hundred boys. Visits occurred approximately every other week. Thirty years later, the youths (who had become adults) were retraced and their criminal records obtained. These records included the violent crimes of assault, attempted assault, kidnapping, robbery, rape, abuse of a female child, weapons charges, manslaughter, intent to murder, or murder. Analyses showed that corporal punishment by their mothers had increased the likelihood of their being convicted for a violent crime even when the punishment was coupled with maternal warmth.

The use of physical punishments to enforce parental demands is likely to legitimize the use of violence (Straus, 1991). In addition, the use of severe punishments has been shown to increase attractiveness of what is protected through punishment. In one of the most famous of the studies demonstrating this phenomenon, children ranked their preferences for five toys. The experimenter placed the toy ranked as second-favorite by the child on a table, telling the child he could play with the other four, but not the one on the table. Half of the children were randomly assigned to each of two conditions. In the "mild threat" condition, the experimenter said he would be annoyed if the child played with the forbidden toy. In the "severe threat" condition, the experimenter said that if the child played with the forbidden toy, the experimenter would be very angry and would take all the toys and never come back. The experimenter left the child for 10 minutes. Approximately 45 days later, the children were again asked to rank the five toys. In the second ranking, 8 of those who were merely told that the experimenter would be annoyed had decreased their preference for the forbidden toy whereas none of the children who were threatened with punishment had they played with the toy decreased their preference for it. Conversely, in the second ranking, 4 of the children from the mild threat condition ranked the forbidden toy as a favorite whereas 14 of those in the severe threat condition regarded the forbidden toy as the favorite. In sum, punishment tended to enhance the value of the forbidden (Aronson and Carlsmith, 1963).

Even those not themselves subjected to violence are affected by exposure to violence (Goldstein & Arms, 1971). Family conflict has long been a reliable predictor of criminal behavior (Emery, 1982; Farrington, 1978, 1986; Hirschi, 1969; Loeber & Stouthamer-Loeber, 1986; McCord, 1982, 1991; Nye, 1957; Power, Ash, Shoenberg, and Sirey, 1974; Rutter, 1971; West & Farrington, 1973). Evidence from a longitudinal study in which children's families were observed over several years and the criminality of the children traced through the adult years suggests that conflict between the parents, is particularly strongly related to violent crimes (McCord, 1979).

Evidence gathered in a study of young children in preschool classrooms suggests a mechanism to account for correlations between exposure to parental conflict and misbehavior. The study showed that occasional exposure to conflict increases cortisol levels, but that exposure to constant stress dampens glucocorticoid responses (Hart, Gunnar, & Cicchetti, 1995). Neuroendocrine activity may be the mechanism by which early stress experiences are linked with a desensitization to the environment that is found among young psychopaths.

Exposure to violence desensitizes witnesses to future violence. For example, Cline, Croft, & Courrier (1973) compared galvanic skin responses and blood volume changes among boys watching nonviolent and violent segments of movies. Those who customarily watched little television showed greater physiological responsiveness to the film segments containing a chase scene and the violent segments of a boxing movie than did the boys who normally watched television more than 25 hours a week. Because there were no differences in physiological responsiveness to a nonviolent ski film or nonviolent segments of the boxing movie, the difference seems to have been induced through exposure. Extending the evidence regarding effects of observing violence, Thomas, Horton, Lippincott, & Drabman (1977) found that watching an aggressive film desensitized children to the distress of a younger child. In this study, children between the ages of 8 and 10 were shown either an aggressive or a nonaggressive film and asked to keep an eye out for a preschool child in the next room. Galvanic skin responses indicated that those watching the aggressive film were less responsive when the child needed help. These studies suggest how exposure to violence affects responses to subsequent stress. The link appears to be through the neuroendocrine system.

Studies of abused children indicate that neuroendocrine responsiveness may have been altered by experiencing maltreatment. As measured by salivary cortisol, maltreated children are less responsive to subsequent stress (Hart, Gunnar, & Cicchetti, 1995).

8. SOCIAL ENVIRONMENT AND VIOLENCE

Apart from conditions of socialization, two environmental factors have been linked with violence: social discrimination and the availability of alcohol. In many societies, groups who are discriminated against tend to have higher rates of criminal violence than those who are better protected by the laws. Within the high risk groups, that is, among the groups who have high rates of violence, victims of discrimination are more likely to be perpetrators of violence. Among blacks reared in Chicago, for example, men who had experienced racial discrimination were more likely to commit violent crimes than were their peers regardless of their childhood aggressiveness (McCord & Ensminger, 1997).

In many societies, as well, violence occurs where and when alcohol is available. There are grounds for attributing some of the coincidence of violence with the use of alcohol to the fact that people who seek excitement are likely to drink in public places, where fights occur. More research is necessary before conclusions regarding causal links between alcohol and violence should be drawn.

9. BUILDING THEORY TO UNDERSTAND PSYCHOPATHIC BEHAVIOR

Understanding psychopathy and violence requires considering individuals as they interact with their environments. In pulling together evidence about psychopathy and violence, I have tried to build a case to explain why psychopaths (or others) choose to commit crimes of violence. In doing so, I am conscious of the requirement that social as well as biological explanations for criminal behavior must leave room for agents to act intentionally.

An adequate theory of intentional action must allow reasons, or motives, to be part of the causal chain of events. To do so, I have developed the Construct Theory. the Construct Theory claims that motivation arises as children are taught to use reasons in justifying actions (McCord, 1997b). Briefly, the Construct Theory claims that motives do not require desires or "wants." The Construct theory regards drives and needs -- at least when conceived to be motivating forces -- as obfuscating fictions. I do not mean that people are never hungry, want sex, and require water -- but rather, that links between hunger and eating, between sexual desire and copulation, between thirst and its quenching are contingent and that particular acts of eating, copulation, and drinking are not adequately explained by reference to putative drives or needs.

Rather than resorting to drives or needs, the Construct Theory considers motives to be supervenient properties of the descriptions linking <u>potentiating reasons</u> to an action. Potentiating reasons serve for actions as arguments do for beliefs. We believe on the basis of convincing arguments, even when what we believe is not what we would like to believe. Similarly, potentiating reasons lead to actions without regard to desires. The degree to which people have potentiating reasons that justify the use of violence varies among individuals and within individuals through time.

The Construct theory of motivation rests on the Fregean idea that language is fundamentally evaluative and public. This position avoids problems tied to theories of action that insist on a chasm between descriptions and evaluations. It also avoids the problems that accrue to theories of language that place meanings in a private realm of images in the mind.

The theory assumes that children learn what to do and what to believe in the process of learning how to use language. Language provides a link between individuals and their societies because concepts are organized by the language in which they can be described. In learning a language, an individual's ideas are constructed in a form that permits their linguistic representation. The Construct theory sees motives as members of a special class of descriptions, as potentiating reasons for action. Understanding why criminals commit particular types of crimes requires understanding why their reasons for action move them to act in antisocial ways.

When children learn a language, they are learning to follow rules, linguistic rules that require complex classifications. To learn a language, children construct categories that they can use to communicate with others in their culture. Sounds acquire meaning in virtue of the rules that permit recognition of repetitions, that enable identification and re-identification of objects and events (Keil, 1994; Nelson, 1996). Children learn not only what to count as tables and chairs, cars and trains, but also what to count as painful or pleasant, undesirable or desirable, and worth avoiding or pursuing. In learning labels, in learning how to name and to re-identify objects and activities, children construct classifications. The classification systems they develop influence what they notice (Keil, 1994; Markman, 1994). The Construct theory adds that the classification system formed through learning language affects how children act as well as what they understand and say.

Learning a language includes learning what J. L. Austin (1962) called "performatives." These are utterances like requesting, apologizing, promising, warning, and advising. In learning language, children learn these activities as well as -- and possibly prior to -- learning how to describe what they see and hear. At very young ages, children in normal settings recognize requests and often do as they are asked. Early in their development, they know that some types of language are grounds for action. In one naturalistic study, the observers found that almost half the toddlers (12 to 15 months in age) complied with their mother's first request to change the course of their actions (Power & Chapieski, 1986). That is, without any overt rewards, children often act because they understand a request.

In recognizing how children learn language, the Construct theory focuses on how what their caregivers do affects what children learn. The theory claims that categories of descriptions form potentiating reasons for an agent to behave in specified ways. Such categories might be labeled, as in a filing system, "to be done" or "to be avoided." Both natural and artificial contingencies inform the child about the world and how to act within it. The studies of babies show that very young children use subtle cues to create their views of the world and how to act within it. This has been demonstrated by studies of neonates who were taught to cry more frequently if their natural cries brought ready response (Hubbard & van IJzendoorn, 1990; Thoman, Korner, & Benson-Williams, 1977).

Studies have shown that by the age of 15 months, infants employ logic in learning language. Markman (1994) discovered that monolingual babies show a preference for having exactly one name for an object. Markman reported a study in which babies were presented with a novel label while holding an object whose name they already knew. The babies looked inside a bucket to find a hidden alternative object to which to attach the name in preference to applying a second name to an already labeled object.

Construct theory explains the fact that different people consider similar events to have different affective characteristics (e.g., as undesirable and desirable) by recognizing that individuals construct different classifications of the events. In infancy and early childhood, caregivers provide the contingencies from which a child learns the category system of his social environment. In teaching children how to act, parents display a variety of cues that indicate the values they themselves place on various grounds for action. Some parents show a child the consequences of misbehavior in terms of how "wrong" actions injure others or objects. These "inductive" measures appear to be particularly effective in reducing the likelihood of future misbehavior (Hoffman, 1977).

Some parents use the word "no," but allow a child to do the act supposedly forbidden -- perhaps following with a punishment. They are teaching the child to use "no" as a sign that something unpleasant might follow. They are also teaching grounds for giving injury. Were they to stop a child's action while saying "no," the child would learn a different meaning for the word.

Dienstbier (1984) describes a study of young, same-sex twins used in a matched-pairs design to evaluate what he and his colleagues considered to be emotion-attribution differences. Each child was placed in a toy room, alone, and asked to watch a miniature slotcar in order to prevent an accident that might destroy the "valuable old" toy. When the child stopped watching the slotcar for a criterion period of time, the car was made to fall (by a hidden observer) and the experimenter returned to the room. One twin in each pair was told that (s)he probably felt unhappy because of what (s)he had done and that those who do the right thing feel good even if no one knows; the other was told that (s)he probably felt unhappy because the experimenter knew what (s)he had done and that those who can show others that they do the right thing feel good. Both were subsequently given new slotcars to watch and allowed to lock their doors so that (they believed) no one would know whether or not they followed instructions to monitor the cars. Out of 12 minutes, the first group failed to watch for 177 seconds whereas the second group failed to watch for 322 seconds, a difference that was highly significant. Although the experimenters inferred emotion as mediating the obtained differences, it should be noted that the information conveyed about what cues to consider salient fits well a picture in which the children in the first (internal attribution) condition were instructed to do the right thing regardless of who might know and the second (external attribution) were informed that what the experimenter might know was the relevant consideration. The experiment did not demonstrate that emotions were involved in the effects; that conclusion depended on the unevaluated assumption that emotions are the foundation for behavior.

When a child is credibly threatened with punishment, the information conveyed extends beyond the intended message that the child ought not do something. A punishment is designed to be unpleasant. Unless the punisher thought it unpleasant, the punishment would not be selected as a means for controlling the child's behavior. What is selected as a punishment, then, shows what is to be considered undesirable.

In addition, the use of punishment and threats of punishment indicate what types of behavior the punisher considers desirable. Punishments are not necessary to stop people from doing what they would not or could not choose to do.

The extent to which preferences can be shaped by the use of punishments and rewards has been demonstrated through arbitrarily arranged activities. Lepper, Sagotsky, Defoe, and Greene (1982) used imaginary foods dubbed "hupe" and "hule." Twenty-eight preschool children were told short stories about Johny or Janie, depending on the sex of the child, being given new foods. For half the children, the mother in the story offered first one and then the other (in counterbalanced order) to the child in the story. For the other half, the mother in the story explained to her child that (s)he could have one ("hupe" or "hule" for different children) if (s)he ate the other. In the contingency condition, where it seemed as though hupe (or hule) was a reward for eating the other, the children judged the second preferable and gave as their reason that the second dish tasted better. No such preference appeared in the noncontingent condition. The effect for preferences under contingency options was replicated with another group of forty children using felt pens and pastels rather than imaginary foods. Thus, the study showed clearly that children can be taught what to value by the nature of choices presented to them.

Identifying something as a reward tends to enhance its value while diminishing that of the rewarded behavior (Boggiano & Main, 1986). Many studies show that rewarding children for performing an activity they already enjoy tends to reduce the children's interest in that activity (e.g., Greene & Lepper, 1974; Lepper, Greene & Nisbett, 1973; Ross, Karniol, & Rothstein, 1976). Outside the laboratory, a study of 72 children between the ages of 7 and 11 years showed that those accustomed to receiving rewards were less likely to be helpful without rewards than were children not accustomed to receiving them (Fabes, Fultz, Eisenberg, May-Plumlee, & Christopher, 1989). In such cases, children have associated receiving rewards with potentiating reasons for doing as they are asked.

The Construct Theory suggests that socialization affects behavior through influencing what counts as a potentiating reason, a reason for action. Once a person develops a set of potentiating reasons, that person will use the set to organize the environment and to act upon it. Therefore, the actions of an individual tend to be predictable. Motivated action, on this theory, is action because of a reason (or set of reasons) and is therefore plausibly considered to be voluntary. The experiences of psychopaths are such as to make it seem reasonable to them to find that many and varied circumstances violence.

10. SUMMARY

In this paper, I have tried to show the multiple ways in which biological characterizations of people are coupled with descriptions of their behavior and attitudes. Whereas studies of psychopaths have sometimes attempted to parse their behavior into biological and sociological components, I have sought to show that this is a mistake. Human behavior affects human biology even as human biology affects behavior. A clear example can be seen in the influence that diet and exercise have on body shape. Ideas influence neural processes even as neural structure can influence ideas, for surely what we experience has some trace in the biological makeup of our minds.

In reviewing socialization practices noted for their influence on children's behavior, I have singled out the deleterious effects of parental neglect and harsh punishments. Such effects are better documented than other, more subtle interactions. They suggest that infants benefit enormously through being reared by caring adults who teach them what behavior is appropriate for the society in which they live.

And finally, I have proposed a theory designed to address some basic issues involved in understanding intentional behavior. If a person's actions are determined through illness, the person would not deserve to be praised or blamed. Intentional behavior is the sort of behavior that deserves reward or punishment.

I have suggested that psychopaths are reared under circumstances that often lead them to choose to act in ways that society finds condemnable. The Construct Theory shows why such behavior can be predictable despite the fact that a psychopath can be held accountable.

REFERENCES

Allen, H. E.; Dinitz, S.; Foster, T. W.; Goldman, H. & Lindner, L. A. (1976): "Sociopathy: An experiment in internal environmental control", *American Behavioral Scientist,* 20 (2), pp. 215-226.

Aronson, E. & Carlsmith, J. M. (1963): "Effect of the severity of threat on the devaluation of forbidden behavior", *Journal of Abnormal and Social Psychology*, 66 (6), pp. 584-588.

Austin, J. L. (1962): *How To Do Things With Words*, Oxford, The Clarendon Press.

Baldwin, D. A. (1991). "Infants' contribution to the achievement of joint reference", *Child Development*, 62, pp. 875-890.

Bender, L. (1947): "Psychopathic behavior disorders in children", in R. Lindner & R. Seliger (Eds.), *Handbook of Correctional Psychology*, New York, Philosophical Library.

Beran, N. J. & Allen, H. E. (1981): "Sociopathic and other mentally ill offenders revisited", in J. L. Barak-Glantz & C. R. Huff (eds.), *The Mad, the Bad, and the Different.*

Berg, N. L. (1974): "Self-concept of neurotic and sociopathic criminal offenders", *Psychological Reports*, 34, p. 622.

Blackburn, R. (1975): "An empirical classification of psychopathic personality", *British Journal of Psychiatry*, 127, pp. 456-460.

Boggiano, A. K. & Main, D. S. (1986): "Enhancing children's interest in activities used as rewards: The bonus effect", *Journal of Personality and Social Psychology*, 31 (6), pp. 1116-1126.

Bowlby, J. (1940): "The influence of early environment on neurosis and neurotic character", *International Journal of Psychoanalysis*, 21, pp. 154-178.

Bowlby, J. (1951): "Maternal care and mental health", *Bulletin of the World Health Organization*, 3, pp. 355-534.

Brennan, P. A.; Mednick, S. A. & Raine, A. (1997): "Biosocial interactions and violence: A focus on perinatal factors", in A. Raine, P. A. Brennan, D. P. Farrington & S. A. Mednick (eds.), *Biosocial Bases of Violence*, New York, Plenum Press, pp. 163-174.

Cairns, R. B.; Cairns, B. D.; Neckerman, H. J.; Ferguson, L. L. & Gariépy, J. L. (1989): "Growth and aggression: I. Childhood to early adolescence", *Developmental Psychology*, 25 (2), pp. 320-330.

Camras, L. A.; Malatesta, C. & Izard, C. E. (1991): "The development of facial expressions in infancy", in R. S. Feldman & B. Rime (eds.), *Fundamentals of Nonverbal Behavior*, New York, Cambridge University Press.

Caspi, A. & Silva, P. A. (1995): "Temperamental Qualities at Age Three Predict Personality Traits in Young Adulthood: Longitudinal Evidence from a Birth cohort", *Child Development*, 66, pp. 486-498.

Cleckley, H. (1941/1976): *The Mask of Sanity*, St. Louis, Mosby.

Cline, V. B.; Croft, R. G. & Courrier, S. (1973): "Desensitization of children to television violence", *Journal of Personality and Social Psychology*, 27 (3), pp. 360-365.

Cloninger, C. R.; Reich, T. & Guze, S. B. (1975): "The multifactorial model of disease transmission: II. Sex differences in the familial transmission of sociopathy", *British Journal of Psychiatry*, 127, pp. 11-22.

Coccaro, E. F. (1995): "The Biology of Aggression", *Science and Medicine*, January/February, 1995, pp. 38-47.

DeCasper, A. J. & Fifer, W. P. (1980): "Of human bonding: Newborns prefer their mothers' voices", *Science*, 208, pp. 1.174-6.

Dienstbier, R. A. (1984): "The role of emotion in moral socialization", in C. E. Izard, J. Kagan & R. B. Zajonc (eds.), *Emotions, Cognitions, & Behavior*, Cambridge University Press.

Dornbusch, S. M.; Carlsmith, J. M.; Bushwall, S. J.; Ritter, P. L.; Leiderman, H.; Hastorf, A. H. & Gross, R. T. (1985): "Single parents, extended households, and the control of adolescents", *Child Development*, 56, pp. 326-341.

Egeland, B. & Sroufe, A. (1981): "Developmental sequelae of maltreatment in infancy", in R. Rizley & D. Cicchetti (eds.), *Developmental Perspectives on Child Maltreatment, New Directions for Child Development*, San Francisco, Jossey-Bass.

Emery, R. E. (1982): "Interparental conflict and the children of discord and divorce", *Psychological Bulletin*, 92, pp. 310-330.

Emmons, T. D. & Webb, W. W. (1974): "Subjective correlates of emotional responsivity and stimulation seeking in psychopaths, normals, and acting-out neurotics", *Journal of Consulting and Clinical Psychology*, 42 (4), p. 620.

Eron, L.; Huesmann, L. R. & Zelli, A. (1991): "The role of parental variables in the learning of aggression", in D. J. Pepler & K. H. Rubin (eds.), *The Development and Treatment of Childhood Aggression*, Hillsdale, Lawrence Erlbaum.

Estabrook, A. H. (1916): *The Jukes in 1915*, Washington, D.C., Carnegie Institution of Washington, #240.

Fabes, Richard A.; Fultz, Jim; Eisenberg, Nancy; May-Plumlee, Traci & Christopher, F. Scott (1989): "Effects of rewards on children's prosocial motivation: A socialization study", *Developmental Psychology*, 25 (4), pp. 509-515.

Farrington, D. P. (1978): "The family backgrounds of aggressive youths", in L. A. Hersov & M. Berger (eds.), *Aggression and antisocial behaviour in childhood and adolescence*, Oxford, Pergamon.

Farrington, D. P. (1986): "Stepping stones to adult criminal careers", in D. Olweus; J. Block & M. Radke-Yarrow (eds.), *Development of Antisocial and Prosocial Behavior*, New York, Academic Press.

Farrington, D. P. (1988): "Social, psychological and biological influences on juvenile delinquency and adult crime", in W. Buikhuisen & S. A. Mednick (eds.), *Explaining Criminal Behaviour: Interdisciplinary Approaches*, New York, E. J. Brill.

Farrington, D. P. (1989): "Early predictors of adolescent aggression and adult violence", *Violence and Victims*, 4 (2), pp. 79-100.

Farrington, D. P. (1992): "Explaining the beginning, progress, and ending of antisocial behavior from birth to adulthood", in J. McCord (ed.), *Facts, Frameworks, and Forecasts: Advances in Criminological Theory*, Vol. 3, New Brunswick, Transaction Press.

Farrington, D. P.; Gundry, G. & West, D. J. (1975): "The familial transmission of criminality", *Medical Science Law*, 15 (3), pp. 177-186.

Ferri, E. (1897): *Criminal Sociology*, New York, D. Appleton & Co.

Field, M. (1940): "Maternal attitudes found in 25 cases of children with primary behavior disorder", *American Journal of Orthopsychiatry*, 10, pp. 293-311.

Fink, A. E. (1938): *Causes of Crime: Biological Theories in the United States 1800-1915*. Philadelphia, PA, University of Pennsylvania Press.

Goldfarb, W. (1945): "Psychological privation in infancy and subsequent adjustment", *American Journal of Orthopsychiatry*, 15, pp. 247-255.

Goldfarb, W. (1958): "Pain reactions in a group of institutionalized schizophrenic children", *American Journal of Orthopsychiatry*, 28, pp. 777-785.

Goldstein, J. H. & Arms, R. L. (1971): "Effects of observing athletic contests on hostility", *Sociometry*, 34 (1), pp. 83-90.

Gough, H. G. (1948): "A sociological theory of psychopathy", *American Journal of Sociology*, 53, pp. 359-366.

Goyer, P. F. & Semple, W. E. (1996): "PET studies of aggression in personality disorder and other nonpsychotic patients", in Stoff, D. M. & Cairns, R. B. (eds.), *Aggression and Violence: Genetic, Neurobiological, and Biosocial Perspectives*, Mahwah, NJ, Lawrence Erlbaum Associates, pp. 219-235.

Greene, David & Lepper, Mark R. (1974): "Effects of extrinsic rewards on children's subsequent intrinsic interest", *Child Development*, 45, pp. 1.141-5.

Greenough, W. T.; Black, J. E. & Wallace, C. S. (1987): "Experience and brain development", *Child Development*, 58, pp. 539-559.

Gunnar, M. R. & Barr, R. G. (1998): "Stress, early brain development, and behavior", *Infants and Young Children*, 11 (1), pp. 1-14.

Gunnar, M. R.; Connors, J. & Isensee, J. (1989): "Lack of stability in neonatal adrenocortical reactivity because of rapid habituation of the adrenocortical response", *Developmental Psychobiology*, 22, pp. 221-233.

Gunnar, M. R.; Hertsgaard, L.; Larson, M. & Rigatuso, J. (1992): "Cortisol and behavioral responses to repeated stressors in the human newborn", *Developmental Psychobiology*, 24, pp. 487-505.

Gunnar-Vongnechten, M. R. (1978): "Changing a frightening toy into a pleasant toy by allowing the infant to control its actions", *Developmental Psychobiology*, 14, pp. 157-162.

Halperin, J. M.; Newcorn, J. H.; Kopstein, I.; McCay, K. E.; Schwartz, S. T.; Stever, L. J. & Sharma, V. (1997): "Serotonin, Aggression, and Parental Psychopathology in Children with Attention-Deficit Hyperactivity Disorder", *Journal of American Academy Child Adolescent Psychiatry*, Vol. 36, No. 10, pp. 1391-1398.

Haller, M. H. (1963/1984): *Eugenics: Hereditarian Attitudes in American Thought*, New Brunswick, Rutgers University Press.

Hare, R. & McPherson, L. M. (1984): "Violent and aggressive behavior by criminal psychopaths", *International Journal of Law and Psychiatry*, 7, pp. 35-50.

Hare, R. D. & Cox, D. N. (1978): "Clinical and empirical conceptions of psychopathy and the selection of subjects for research", in R. D. Hare & D. Schalling (eds.), *Psychopathic Behaviour*, Chichester, John Wiley & Sons.

Hare, R. D. (1970): *Psychopathy: Theory and Research*, New York, John Wiley & Sons.

Hare, R. D. (1978): "Electrodermal and cardiovascular correlates of psychopathy", in R. D. Hare & D. Schalling (eds.), *Psychopathic Behaviour*, Chichester, John Wiley & Sons.

Hare, R. D. (1990): "A research scale for the assessment of psychopathy in criminal populations", *Personality and Individual Differences*, 1, pp. 11-119.

Harper, M. A.; Morris, M. & Bleyerveld, J. (1972): "The significance of an abnormal EEG in psychopathic personalities", *Australian & New Zealand Journal of Psychiatry*, 6, pp. 215-224.

Harris, G. T.; Rice, M. E. & Cormier, C.A. (1991): "Psychopathy and violent recidivism", *Law and Human Behavior*, 15, 6, pp. 625-639.

Hart, J.; Gunnar, M. R. & Cicchetti, D. (1995): "Salivary cortisol in maltreated children: Evidence of relations between neuroendocrine activity and social competence", *Development and Psychopathology*, 7, pp. 11-26.

Hawkins, J. D.; Herrenkohl, T.; Farrington, D. P.; Brewer, D.; Catalano, R. F. & Harachi, T. W. (1998): "A review of predictors of youth violence", in R. Loeber & D. P. Farrington (eds.), *Serious & Violent Juvenile Offenders*, Thousand Oaks, Sage Publications.

Herrenkohl, R. C. & Herrenkohl, E. C. (1981): "Some antecedents and developmental consequences of child maltreatment", in R. Risley & D. Cicchetti (eds.), *Developmental Perspectives on Child Maltreatment*, San Francisco, Jossey-Bass.

Hinton, J.; O'Neill, M.; Hamilton, S. & Burke, M. (1980): "Psychophysiological differentiation between psychopathic and schizophrenic abnormal offenders", *British Journal of Social and Clinical Psychology*, 19 (3), pp. 257-269.

Hirschi, T. (1969): *Causes of Delinquency*, Berkeley, University of California Press.

Hoffman, M. (1977): "Moral internalization: Current Theory and research", in L. Berkowitz (ed.), *Advances in Experimental Social Psychology*, New York, Academic Press.

Hubbard, F. O. A. & van Izendoorn, M. H. (1990): "Responsiveness to infant crying: Spoiling or comforting the baby? A descriptive longitudinal study in a normal Dutch sample", in W. Koops, H. J. G. Soppe, J. L. van der Linden, P. C. M. Molenaar, & J. J. F. Schroots (eds.), *Developmental Psychology behind the dikes: An outline of developmental psychological research in the Netherlands*, Delft, Uitgeverij Eburon.

Kandel, E. R. & Mednick, S. A. (1991): "Perinatal complications predict violent offending", *Criminology*, 29(3), pp. 519-529.

Karli, P. (1996): "The brain and socialization: a two-way mediation across the life course", in Magnusson, D. (ed.), *The Lifespan Development of Individuals: Behavioral, neurobiological, and psychosocial perspectives*, Cambridge, England, Cambridge University Press, pp. 341-356.

Karpman, B. (1941): "On the need of separating Psychopathy into two distinct clinical types: The symptomatic and the idiopathic", *Journal of Criminal Psychopathology*, 3 (July), pp. 112-137.

Kavanagh, K. A.; Youngblade, L.; Reid, J. B. & Fagot, B. I. (1988): "Interactions between children and abusive versus control parents", *Journal of Clinical Child Psychology*, 17 (2), pp. 137-142.

Keil, F. C. (1994): "Explanation, association, and the acquisition of word meaning", in L. Gleitman & B. Landau (eds.), *The Acquisition of the Lexicon*, Cambridge, MA, The MIT Press.

Klinteberg, B. A. F.; Humble, K. & Schalling, D. (1992): "Personality and Psychopathy of Males with a History of Early Criminal Behaviour", *European Journal of Personality*, 6 (4), pp. 245-266.

Knoblich, G. & King, R. (1991): "Biological correlates of criminal behavior", in J. McCord (ed.), *Facts, Frameworks, and Forecasts: Advances in Criminological Theory, Vol. 3* (1-21), New Brunswick, Transaction Press.

Laub, J. H. & Sampson, R. J. (1988): "Unraveling families and delinquency: A reanalysis of the Gluecks' data", *Criminology*, 26 (3), pp. 355-380.

Lepper, Mark R.; Greene, David & Nisbett, Robert E. (1973): "Undermining children's intrinsic interest with extrinsic rewards", *Journal of Personality and Social Psychology*, 28 (1), pp. 129-137.

Lepper, Mark R.; Sagotsky, Gerald; Dafoe, Janet L. & Greene, David (1982): "Consequences of superfluous social constraints: Effects on young children's social influences and subsequent intrinsic interest", *Journal of Personality and Social Psychology*, 41 (1), pp. 51-65.

Levy, D. (1937): "Primary affect hunger", *American Journal of Psychiatry*, 94, pp. 643-652.

Liska, A. E. & Reed, M. D. (1985): "Ties to conventional institutions and delinquency: Estimating reciprocal effects", *American Sociological Review*, 50 (August), pp. 547-560.

Loeber, R. & Stouthamer-Loeber, M. (1986): "Family factors as correlates and predictors of juvenile conduct problems and delinquency", in M. Tonry & N. Morris (eds.), *Crime and Justice*, Vol. 7, Chicago, University of Chicago Press.

Lombroso, C. (1896/1911): *Criminal Man*, in Gina Lombroso-Ferrero (ed.), Boston, G. P. Putnam.

Lykken, D. T. (1957): "A study of anxiety in the sociopathic personality", *Journal of Abnormal and Social Psychology*, 55 (1), pp. 6-10.

Lynam, D. R. (1996): "Early Identification of Chronic Offenders: Who is the Fledgling Psychopath?", *Psychological Bulletin*, vol. 120, No. 2, pp. 209-234.

Lynam, D. R. (1997): "Pursuing the Psychopath: Capturing the Fledgling Psychopath in a Nomological Net", *Journal of Abnormal Psychology*, Vol. 106, No. 3, pp. 425-438.

Magnusson, D.; Klinteberg, B. A. F. & Stattin, H. (1992): "Autonomic activity/reactivity, behavior and crime in a longitudinal perspective", in J. McCord (ed.), *Facts, Frameworks, and Forecasts: Advances in Criminological Theory*, Vol. 3, New Brunswick, Transaction Press.

Main, M. & Goldwyn, R. (1984): "Predicting rejection of her infant from mother's representation of her own experience: Implications for the abused-abusing intergenerational cycle", *Child Abuse & Neglect*, 8 (2), pp. 203-217.

Mannuzza, S.; Klein, R. G.; Konig, P. H. & Giampino, T. L. (1989): "Hyperactive boys almost grown up: IV. Criminality and its relationship to psychiatric status", *Archives of General Psychiatry*, 46 (12), pp. 1.073-9.

Markman, E. M. (1994): "Constraints on word meaning in early language acquisition", in L. Gleitman & B. Landau (eds.), *The Acquisition of the Lexicon*, Cambridge, MA, The MIT Press.

McCord, J & Ensminger, M. E. (1997): "Multiple risks and comorbidity in an African-American population", *Criminal Behaviour and Mental Health*, 7, pp. 339-352.

McCord, J. (1979): "Some child-rearing antecedents of criminal behavior in adult men", *Journal of Personality and Social Psychology*, 37, pp. 1.477-86.

McCord, J. (1982): "A longitudinal view of the relationship between paternal absence and crime", in J. Gunn & D. P. Farrington (eds.), *Abnormal offenders, delinquency, and the criminal justice system*, Chichester, Wiley.

McCord, J. (1983): "A forty year perspective on effects of child abuse and neglect", *Child Abuse and Neglect*, 7, pp. 265-270.

McCord, J. (1991): "The cycle of crime and socialization practices", *Journal of Criminal Law and Criminology*, 82 (1), pp. 211-228.

McCord, J. (1997a): "On Discipline", *Psychological Inquiry*, 8 (3), pp. 215-217.

McCord, J. (1997b). "He Did It Because He Wanted To...", in W. Osgood (ed.), *Nebraska Symposium on Motivation*, Vol. 44, Lincoln NE, University of Nebraska Press.

McCord, Joan (1991): "Family relationships, juvenile delinquency, and adult criminality", *Criminology*, 29 (3), pp. 397-417.

McCord, W. & McCord, J. (1964): *The Psychopath: An essay on the criminal mind*, New York, Van Nostrand Reinhold.

Mednick, S. A. (1977): "A bio-social theory of the learning of law-abiding behavior", in S. A. Mednick & K. O. Christiansen (eds.), *Biosocial Bases of Criminal Behavior*, New York, Gardner.

Moffitt, T. E. (1997): "Neuropsychology, Antisocial Behavior, and Neighborhood Context", in J. McCord (ed.), *Violence and Childhood in the Inner City*, New York, Cambridge University Press, pp. 116-170.

Moffitt, T.; Caspi, A.; Fawcett, P.; Brammer, G. L.; Raleigh, M.; Yuwiler, A. & Silva, P. (1997): "Whole blood serotonin and family background relate to male violence", in A. Raine, P. A. Brennan, D. P. Farrington & S. A. Mednick (eds.), *Biosocial Bases of Violence*, New York, Plenum Press, pp. 231-249.

Morel, B. A. (1857): *Traité des Dégénérescence Physiques, Intellectuelles et Morales de L'Espèce Humaine*, Paris.

Nelson, K. (1996): *Language in Cognitive Development: Emergence of the Mediated Mind*, Cambridge, England, Cambridge University Press.

Newell, H. W. (1934): "The Psycho-dynamics of Maternal Rejection", *American Journal of Orthopsychiatry*, 4, pp. 387-401.

Newell, H. W. (1936): "A Further Study of Maternal Rejection", *American Journal of Orthopsychiatry*, 6, pp. 576-589.

Nye, F.I. (1957): "Child adjustment in broken and in unhappy unbroken homes", *Marriage and Family Living*, 19, pp. 356-361.

Olds, D. L.; Henderson, C. R.; Cole, R.; Eckenrode, J; Kitzman, H.; Luckey, D.; Pettitt, L.; Sidora, K.; Morris, P. & Powers, J. (1998): "Long-term effects of nurse home visitation on children's criminal and antisocial behavior: 15-year follow-up of a randomized controlled trial", *Journal of the American Medical Association*, 280, pp. 1238-1244.

Olweus, D. (1979): "Stability of aggressive patterns in males: A review", *Psychological Bulletin*, 86 (4), pp. 852-875.

Olweus, D. (1980). "Familial and temperamental determinants of aggressive behavior in adolescent boys: A causal analysis", *Developmental Psychology*, 16, pp. 644-660.

Partridge, G. E. (1928): "A Study of 50 Cases of Psychopathic Personality", *American Journal of Psychiatry*, 7, pp. 953-973.

Perry, D. G. & Perry, L. C. (1974): "Denial of suffering in the victim as a stimulus to violence in aggressive boys", *Child Development*, 45 (1), pp. 55-62.

Pine, D. S., Wasserman, G. A., Coplan, J., Fried, J. a., Huang, Y. Y., Kassir, S., Greenhill, L., Shaffer, D., Parsons, B. (1996): "Platelet Serotonin 2A (5-HT2a) Receptor Characteristics and Parenting Factors for Boys at Risk for Delinquency: A Preliminary Report", *American Journal Psychiatry* Vol. 153, No 4, pp. 538-544.

Pinel, P. (1806/1962): *A Treatise on Insanity*, New York, Hafner Publishing Co.

Power, M. J.; Ash, P. M.; Shoenberg, E. & Sirey, E. C. (1974): "Delinquency and the family", *British Journal of Social Work*, 4, pp. 13-38.

Power, T. G. & Chapieski, M. L. (1986): "Childrearing and impulse control in toddlers: A naturalistic investigation", *Developmental Psychology*, 22 (2), pp. 271-275.

Prichard, J. C. (1837/1973): *A Treatise on Insanity and Other Disorders Affecting the Mind*, New York, Arno Press.

Pulkkinen, L. & Tremblay, R. E. (1992): "Patterns of boys' social adjustment in two cultures and at different ages: A longitudinal perspective", *International Journal of Behavioral Development*, 15 (4), pp. 527-553.

Quay H. C. (1977): "Psychopathic behavior: Reflections on its nature, origins, and treatment", in F. Weizmann & I. Uzgiris (eds.), *The Structuring of Experience*, New York, Plenum.

Raine, A. (1996): "Autonomic nervous system activity and violence", in Stoff, D. M. & Cairns, R. B. (eds.), *Aggression and Violence: Genetic, Neurobiological, and Biosocial Perspectives*, Mahway, NJ, Lawrence Erlbaum Associates, pp. 145-168.

Raine, A. (1996a): "Autonomic nervous system factors underlying disinhibited, antisocial, and violent behavior: Biosocial perspectives and treatment implications", in C. F. Ferris & T. Grisso (eds), *Understanding Aggressive Behavior in Children, Vol. 794, Annals of the New York Academy of Sciences*, Sept. 20, pp. 46-59.

Riese, M. L. (1990): "Neonatal temperament in monozygotic and dizygotic twin pairs", *Child Development*, 61(4), pp. 1230-1237.

Robins, L. N. (1966): *Deviant Children Grown Up*, Baltimore, Williams & Wilkins.

Ross, M.; Karniol, R. & Rothstein, M. (1976): "Reward contingency and intrinsic motivation in children: A test in the delay of gratification hypothesis", *Journal of Personality and Social Psychology*, 33, pp. 442-447.

Rotenberg, M. (1978): "Psychopathy and differential insensitivity", in R. D. Hare & D. Schalling (eds.), *Psychopathic Behaviour*, Chichester, John Wiley & Sons.

Rutter, M. (1971): "Parent-child separation: Psychological effects on the Children", *Journal of Child Psychology and Psychiatry*, 12, pp. 233-260.

Rutter, M. (1972): *Maternal Deprivation Reassessed*, Middlesex, England, Penguin.

Sagi, A. & Hoffman, M. L. (1976): "Empathic distress in the newborn", *Developmental Psychology*, 12 (2), pp. 175-176.

Satterfield, J. H. (1987): "Childhood diagnostic and neurophysiological predictors of teenage arrest rates: An eight-year prospective study", in S. A. Mednick, T. E. Moffitt & S. A. Stack (eds.), *The Causes of Crime: New Biological Approaches*, Cambridge, Cambridge University Press.

Schaal, B. (1988): "Olfaction in infants and children: developmental and functional perspectives", *Chemical Senses*, 13 (2), pp. 145-190.

Schalling, D. (1978): "Psychopathy-related personality variables and the psychophysiology of socialization", in R. D. Hare & D. Schalling (eds.), *Psychopathic Behaviour*, Chichester, John Wiley & Sons.

Schmauk, F. J. (1970): "Punishment, arousal, and avoidance learning in sociopaths", *Journal of Abnormal Psychology*, 76 (3), pp. 325-335.

Schuckit, M. A. (1973): "Alcoholism and sociopathy--Diagnostic Confusion", *Quarterly Journal of Studies on Alcohol*, 34, pp. 157-164.

Schulsinger, F. (1977): "Psychopathy: Heredity and environment", in S. A. Mednick & K. O. Christiansen (eds.), *Biosocial Bases of Criminal Behavior*, New York, Gardner.

Siddle, D.A.T. (1977): "Electrodermal activity and psychopathy", in S. A. Mednick & K. O. Christiansen (eds.), *Biosocial Bases of Criminal Behavior*, New York, Gardner.

Siegel, R. A. (1978): "Probability of punishment and suppression of behavior in psychopathic and nonpsychopathic offenders", *Journal of Abnormal Psychology*, 87 (5), pp. 514-522.

Simner, M. L. (1971): "Newborn's response to the cry of another infant", *Developmental Psychology*, 5, pp. 136-150.

Snyder, H. N. (1998): "Appendix: - Serious, violent, and chronic juvenile offenders -- an assessment of the extent of and trends in officially recognized serious criminal behavior in a delinquent population", in R. Loeber & D. P. Farrington (eds.), *Serious & Violent Juvenile Offenders*, Thousand Oaks, Sage Publications.

Spence, M. J. & DeCasper, A. J. (1987): "Prenatal experience with low-frequency maternal-voice sounds influences neonatal perception of maternal voice samples", *Infant Behavior and Development*, 10, pp. 133-142.

Spielberger, C. D.; Kling, J. K. & O'Hagan, S. E. J. (1978): "Dimensions of psychopathic personality: Antisocial behavior and anxiety", in R. D. Hare & D. Schalling (eds.), *Psychopathic Behaviour*, Chichester, John Wiley & Sons.

Stattin, H. & Magnusson, D. (1989): "The role of early aggressive behavior in the frequency, seriousness, and type of later crime", *Journal of Consulting and Clinical Psychology*, 57 (6), pp. 710-718.

Straus, M. A. (1991): "Discipline and deviance: Physical punishment of children and violence and other crime in adulthood", *Social Problems*, 38 (2) (May), pp. 133-154.

Symonds, P. M. (1939): *The Psychology of Parent-Child Relations*, New York, D. Appleton-Century Co.

Thoman, E. B.; Korner, A. F. & Benson-Williams, L. (1977): "Modification of responsiveness to maternal vocalization in the neonate", *Child Development*, 48, pp. 563-569.

Thomas, M. H.; Horton, R. W.; Lippincott, E. C. & Drabman, R. S. (1977): "Desensitization to portrayals of real-life aggression as a function of exposure to television violence", *Journal of Personality and Social Psychology*, 35, pp. 450-458.

Tremblay, R. (1991): "Commentary: Aggression, prosocial behavior, and gender. Three magic words but no magic wand", in D. Pepler & K. Rubin (eds.), *The Development and Treatment of Childhood Aggression*, Hillsdale, NJ, Lawrence Erlbaum.

Wadsworth, M. E. J. (1976): "Delinquency, pulse rates and early emotional deprivation", *The British Journal of Criminology*, 16 (3), pp. 245-256.

Weiss, B.; Dodge, K. A.; Bates, J. E. & Pettit, G. S. (1992): "Some consequences of early harsh discipline: Child aggression and a maladaptive social information processing style", *Child Development*, 63, pp. 1321-1335.

Wells, L. E. & Rankin, J. H. (1988): "Direct parental controls and delinquency", *Criminology*, 26 (2), pp. 263-285.

West, D. J. & Farrington, D. P. (1973): *Who Becomes Delinquent?*, London, Heinemann.

Widom, C. S. (1989): "Child abuse, neglect, and violent criminal behavior", *Criminology*, 27 (2), pp. 251-271.

Wolman, B. B. (1987): *The Sociopathic Personality*, New York, Brunner/Mazel.

Zuckerman, M. (1978): "Sensation seeking and psychopathy", in R. D. Hare & D. Schalling (eds.), *Psychopathic Behaviour*, Chichester

Chapter 9

IS EFFECTIVE TREATMENT OF PSYCHOPATHY POSSIBLE?

What We Know and What We Need to Know

Friedrich Lösel
Institute of Psychology, University of Erlangen-Nuremberg, Germany

1. INTRODUCTION

Psychopaths represent a major challenge for the criminal justice system in democratic societies. With such persons, it is particularly difficult to find a balance between the aims of just punishment, the safety of society, and rehabilitation. Whereas the first two aims are widely accepted for offenders with psychopathic personality, there is much skepticism regarding rehabilitation or treatment. Successful therapeutic modification of human behavior requires an emotional bond between the therapist and the client, cooperation, openness, expressiveness, reciprocal affirmation, and an adequate duration of treatment (Orlinsky, Grawe, & Parks, 1994). However, it is exactly these criteria that psychopaths do not fulfill (Cleckley, 1976; Hare, 1993). Their grandiose sense of self-worth and lack of remorse act against any real motivation to change. Pathological lying disrupts honest communications within therapy. Shallow affect as well as callousness and lack of empathy impede serious work on emotions in social relationships. Glibness and manipulative behavior lead to superficial role play and deception instead of true cooperation. As a consequence, psychosocial interventions are often broken off or have no effect (Blackburn, 1993; Hare, 1995; Lösel, 1998).

However, we must differentiate cautiously between empirical knowledge and a basic assumption that psychopaths are untreatable. Although forensic experts agree that we do not yet possess optimal measures for managing and (perhaps) treating psychopaths, most of them do not conclude that nothing can be done (e.g., Tennent, Tennent, Prins, & Bedford, 1993). Even from a very cautious and not naively optimistic perspective, there are many arguments for increasing our efforts toward adequate programs for psychopaths. For example:

1.1. The lack of empirically sound studies

Although many articles have dealt with the treatment of psychopathy, there is a clear deficit of well-controlled research in this field (Lösel, 1998). Only a handful of treatment evaluations address psychopaths who are assessed precisely with the Psychopathy Checklist-Revised (PCL-R; Hare, 1991) or related instruments. The vast majority of studies refer to criminality in general; others, to legal definitions of psychopathy or broader concepts of antisocial personality. Quasi-experimental control-group studies on offender treatment mainly address juveniles in community or institutional settings. There is far less controlled treatment research on personality-disordered adults in prisons or forensic hospitals in which it is particularly difficult to recruit equivalent comparison groups.

1.2. Safety of society

Although the prevalence of psychopaths varies between cultures (Cooke, 1998), they form a substantial proportion of serious and persistent offenders. In North America, for example, approximately 28% of prisoners have a PCL score of 30 or above (Hare, 1991). In Europe, corresponding rates are much lower (Cooke, 1998), although we still found approximately 12% in Bavarian prisons (Bender & Lösel, 1999). As several cohort studies have shown, persistent offenders such as psychopaths are responsible for more than 50% of the officially recorded offenses in each age group (Loeber, Farrington, & Waschbusch, 1998). Thus, relatively effective treatment of psychopaths could contribute to a substantial reduction of crime rates in societies. This argument holds for the majority of cases in which the crimes committed are not so serious as to result in life-time prison sentences.

1.3. Management of institutions

Psychopaths often exhibit institutional misbehavior, aggression, and other disciplinary problems (Coid, 1998; Rice, Harris, & Cormier, 1992; Salekin, Rogers, & Sewell, 1996). Their verbal aggression, intimidation, negative comparisons, accusation of others, demand for trust, purposeful misinterpretations, exaggerations, lying, playing for sympathy, and other psychopathic behavior contribute to institutional conflicts and a negative climate (Doren, 1987). Therefore, relatively successful treatment is not only in the interest of rehabilitation for these inmates but also good for the social climate and regime of the whole institution.

1.4. Problems of classification

As Harris, Rice, and Quinsey (1994) and others have shown, there is evidence that psychopathy can be conceptualized as a taxon. On the other hand, the cultural differences in mean scores and item characteristics of the PCL-R (Cooke, 1998) question the existence of one exact cutting point for classification. This is in line with dimensional concepts of psychopathy (e.g., Blackburn & Coid, 1998; Livesley, 1998). We cannot discuss the pros and cons for both positions here. However, if we are still unable to definitely decide about this issue, we also cannot conclude whether a person with a specific score is untreatable or not. Because we also have to take manifold individual features and comorbidies into account, it is adequate to assume more or less graded differences in treatability than a clear cutting point.

1.5. Moderate predictive validity

Psychopathy and particularly the PCL-R and its derivates are among the best predictors of violent and other kinds of recidivism (Hart, 1998; Hemphill, Hare & Wong, 1998; Salekin et al., 1996). Typical prospective correlations are approximately .30 plus/minus .10. These small to moderate correlations are partially due to the single-act criterion of reoffending, problems with its official definition, and other methodological reasons. On the other hand, the large amount of unexplained variance indicates general limits in predicting human behavior and basic aspects of developmental flexibility (Lösel & Bender, in press). However, if psychopathy is only partially relevant for criminal development, we cannot conclude that correctional treatment of this group will fail in principle.

1.6. Biosocial interactions

Research suggests that there are strong biological and probably genetic bases of persistent antisociality and psychopathy (Rowe, 1994; Raine, 1993). In superficial discussions, such results are often misunderstood as an argument for untreatability. However, biological dispositions and heritability never mean that behavior cannot be modified. The genetic information sets only the reaction norm for the phenotype. As phenylketonuria and various other diseases demonstrate, even a clearly genetic defect can be more or less compensated by appropriate educational and social influences. Similarly, antisocial behavior must be understood as outcome of complex developmental pathways and interactions betweeen biological and social factors (Lösel & Bender, in press; Raine et al., 1997).

1.7. Progress in basic research

A lot of literature on the treatment of psychopaths was written before the

1980s. At this time, however, we did not know very much about this disorder (Hare, 1995; 1998). It is only during the last two decades, that our knowledge on the assessment, classification, etiology, and prediction, as well as the biological cognitive, emotional, and behavioral correlates of psychopathy has increased substantially. Progress in basic research is a necessary condition for the development of successful techniques. Insofar, deficits in the area of treatment for psychopathy may be interpreted as a more or less normal delay between basic research and technological application. History is full of examples of how formerly "untreatable" diseases and disorders became relatively controllable after breakthroughs in basic knowledge.

1.8. Progress in research on offender treatment

The situation in psychopathy treatment is similar to that in general offender rehabilitation some time ago. During the 1970s, and still in the 1990s, we find skepticism that is summarized in the "nothing works" doctrine (Logan et al., 1991; Martinson, 1974). A substantial increase in studies, theoretical advances in programming, controlled evaluation designs, and, in particular, systematic meta-analytic integrations of research have led to more differentiated perspectives (Hollin, 1999; Lösel, 1995a). There is now consistent evidence for an overall positive effect and substantial outcome differences between modes of treatment and other moderating factors such as setting, offender groups, program integrity, and so forth. Thus, the discussion has changed from "nothing works" to "what works."

1.9. Realistic expectations of efficacy

In the treatment of seriously antisocial behavior, we cannot expect "big bang" effects. Difficulties of program implementation, multiply disordered clients, low treatment motivation, counteracting factors of prisonization, small sample sizes, problems of outcome measurement, and other factors contribute to small and often non-significant results (Lösel, 1995). Insofar, evaluations of psychopathy treatment should be based on realistic expectations. However, even small effects may have practical significance and be cost-effective (Prentky, & Burgess, 1995; Welsh & Farrington, 2000). The situation is similar to other very difficult areas of treatment such as alcohol and drug abuse. Although, for a long time, progress was only slow in these fields, the necessity of treatment was never questioned in principle.

1.10. Avoidance of negative effects

Discussions on the treatment of psychopaths focus mainly on positive effects. However, some data suggest that therapy may make psychopaths even worse (Rice et al., 1992). Perhaps, some types of programs merely provide the psychopath with better ways of manipulating, deceiving, and abusing people (Hare, 1993). Some negative outcomes are also reported from treatment and prevention in juvenile offenders (Lipsey & Wilson, 1998; McCord, 1978). Therefore, increased evaluation is necessary not only to improve our knowledge about what works but also to avoid inadequate reactions that may have a detrimental effect.

Based on these and other reasons, the following section will briefly address the results of offender treatment research and, in particular, outcomes in psychopathic groups.

2. RESULTS OF TREATMENT EVALUATION

During the last 15 years, a number of meta-analyses have integrated more than 600 relatively well-controlled studies on offender treatment (Hollin, 1999; Lösel, 1995a). The types of offenders, modes of treatment, settings, program duration, follow-up periods, outcome measures, and other characteristics of the design of the single studies are rather different. However, the overall result is relatively similar: In comparison with untreated control groups, treated offenders show less recidivism or otherwise positive outcomes. Depending on computation and weighting methods, mean effect sizes (expressed as correlation coefficient *phi*) vary between .05 (Lipsey, 1992a) and .21 (Redondo, Sanchez-Meca, & Garrido, in press). The general mean *ES* is approximately .10 plus/minus .05 (Lösel, 1995a). Thus, if the recidivism rate in the control group is 50%, the rate in the treated group is 10 percentage points less. In addition to this overall positive outcome, meta-analyses suggest relatively consistent differences between various modes of treatment. In the following, I shall discuss results on four principal approaches: (a) programs that contain psychotherapy, behavior modification, education, and related psychosocial intervention; (b) more complex designs of the whole context such as therapeutic communities, milieu therapy, and social therapy; (c) traditional criminal justice reactions that focus on punishment and deterrence; and (d) pharmacological treatment of antisocial behavior.

2.1. Psychotherapeutic, educational, and related programs

Various meta-analyses confirm that theoretically well-founded, multimodal, cognitive-behavioral therapy and educational programs show effects that are substantially larger than the mean *ES* (e.g., Andrews et al., 1990; Gendreau & Goggin, 1996; Gendreau & Ross, 1987; Lipsey, 1992a; Lipsey & Wilson, 1998; Redondo et al., 1999). In community treatment of serious juvenile offenders, family oriented programs also seem to be promising (Lipsey & Wilson, 1998). The most effective types of program include elements that address cognitive restructuring, problem-solving, self-control, anger management, victim empathy, and social skills training (e.g., Ross, Fabiano, & Ross, 1995). In contrast, low-structured, psychodynamic, or nondirective therapy, unspecific case work and counseling, primarily deterrent measures such as boot camps, or diversion without psychosocial components are overall less effective. The outcome differences between various modes of treatment should not be used as an argument in the traditional rivalry between "schools" of psychotherapy. Labels such as "behavioral," "cognitive-behavioral," "psychodynamic," and so forth can be rather superficial and often are not validated in process analyses of the respective treatment. For example, whereas overall "behavioral" programs are evaluated as relatively successful in meta-analyses on juvenile offender treatment (Lipsey, 1992), operant techniques such as token economies show no long-term effects on antisocial behavior (Rutter, Giller, & Hagell, 1998), and mainly aversive techniques even exhibit negative outcomes in sex offender treatment (Hall, 1995). Instead of broad labels, we need to compare the specific content of procedures that may overlap between different basic orientations. Even well-known psychoanalysts, for example, have not recommended their classical therapy, but structured and educational approaches when treating antisocial behavior (Aichhorn, 1925; Eissler, 1949). Basic concepts of theoretically and empirically well-founded offender treatment seem to be more adequate than traditional "schools" of psychotherapy. For example, appropriate programs should at least meet three principles (Andrews et al., 1990): (a) The level of service should be matched to the risk of clients (risk principle). (b) The targets of services should be matched to the specific criminogenic needs of the offenders (need principle). (c) Styles and modes of service should be matched to the respective learning styles and abilities of offenders (responsivity principle). Programs that meet these three principles are often, but not necessarily, based on cognitive-behavioral concepts. They produce *ES*s from .20 to .30; that is more than twice the general average (Andrews et al., 1990; Gendreau & Goggin, 1996). Programs that do not realize such principles show weaker or sometimes even negative effects.

Overall, cognitive-behavioral, multimodal and related concepts of appropriate offender treatment are relatively successful in groups of serious and violent offenders that may contain a substantial proportion of psychopaths. The same type of program also shows relatively positive outcomes with sexual offenders (e.g., Hall, 1995; Lösel, in press; Marshall, Fernandez, Hudson, & Ward, 1998). Modifying thinking patterns, improving skills, and encouraging self-control can lead to a noncriminal lifestyle without changing the basic personality dispositions that are most difficult to modify. Therefore, these approaches may also be the most adequate ones for psychopaths. This is supported by a meta-analysis from Esteban, Garrido, and Molero (1995). In this study, offenders with antisocial or psychopathic personality disorder showed the worst outcomes overall in any type of treatment program. However, these differences were the smallest for cognitive-behavioral programs.

2.2. Therapeutic communities, milieu therapy, and social therapy

The focus of these modes of treatment is not a single and separate program but the institutional and social context as a whole. They normally contain some of the therapeutic programs mentioned above. Therapeutic communities (TCs) and similar approaches try to (a) establish a more humane and informal climate than in traditional correctional institutions; (b) transfer more responsibilities to the inmates; (c) promote therapeutic and supportive group processes; and (d) strengthen interchanges with the community in the areas of work, education, leisure activities, and social relations (e.g., Genders & Player, 1995; Roberts, 1997).

There are fewer controlled studies on these complex modes of treatment than on the more specific programs. Because TC and other social-therapeutic approaches mainly address serious offenders in institutional settings, it is rather difficult to form equivalent control groups that do not receive any kind of treatment. Particularly in clinical settings, important research has not been able to include control groups (e.g., Dolan, 1997; Robertson & Gunn, 1987). A number of studies show that TCs have a positive impact on psychiatric symptoms, attitudinal conformity, personal responsibility, and variables such as locus of control (e.g., Cullen, 1997; Dolan, Evans, & Wilson, 1992; Genders & Player, 1995; Gunn et al., 1978; McCord, 1982). These therapeutic regimes are also accompanied by a better institutional climate and fewer problems with difficult offenders (e.g., Cooke, 1989; Cullen, 1994; Ortmann, 2000; Peat & Winfree, 1992). With respect to recidivism, however, a differentiated view is necessary. Relatively low structured, self-governing, and permissive TCs and milieu therapy seem to have no general positive effect on reoffending (e.g., Andrews et al., 1990; McCord, 1982; Wexler, Falkin, & Lipton, 1990). Results are better for more hierarchical TCs and social-therapeutic prisons with a clear structure of time, work, and roles; reinforcement of good conduct by assigning greater responsibilities; sequential interactions with the outside world, and so forth (e.g. Lösel & Egg, 1997; Ortmann, 2000; Wexler et al., 1990). In the latter institutions, the overall *ES* is approximately .10 or .15 (Lösel, 1995b). Although this is less than the most appropriate single programs mentioned above, it has to be taken into account that we are dealing often with particularly high-risk offenders.

Psychopathic offenders also benefit least from TC and related complex modes of treatment (e.g., Dolan, 1997; Esteban et al., 1995; Harris, Rice, & Cormier, 1991; Ogloff, Wong, & Greenwood, 1990; Reiss, Grubin, & Meux, 1999; Robertson & Gunn, 1987). This is particularly the case for low-structured regimes. Under these conditions, psychopaths may even show worse outcomes than untreated offenders (e.g., Rice et al., 1992). These and other results indicate again that broad program labels can be misleading. Whereas some forms of TC may be counterproductive for psychopathic offenders, clearly structured, hierarchical, responsibility-oriented regimes are more promising. As for drug-addicted offenders or sex offenders, adequate TCs should also be complemented by structured programs of aftercare and relapse prevention (Cullen, 1997; Laws, 1999; Serin, 1995; Wexler, 1997).

2.3. Measures of punishment and deterrence

Because treatment programs for offenders often are delivered within prison or other custodial contexts, there are partial confounds with measures of punishment and deterrence. Furthermore, punishment is an established principle of behavior modification and thus a potential mode of treatment (Brennan & Mednick, 1994). Insofar, the programs we are addressing under the label of "punishment" should not be viewed as being totally different from any kind of treatment approaches.

Several meta-analyses have found that pure measures of punishment or deterrence show weak effects or even sometimes negative effects on recidivism (e.g., Andrews et al., 1990; Lipsey, 1992a; Lipsey & Wilson, 1998; Redondo et al., 1999). Intensive probation supervision programs, "punishment smarter" programs and other forms of alternative sanctioning also do not seem to be more effective (Gendreau, Paparozzi, Little, & Goddard, 1993; Junger-Tas, 1993; Petersilia, Turner, & Dechenes, 1992). Gendreau and Goggin (1996) performed separate comparisons of the evaluations of incarceration, intermitted incarceration, restitution, scared straight programs, electronic monitoring, drug testing, and fines. Only the restitution programs showed a small positive *ES*.

These and other findings question whether the merely formal variation of criminal justice measures and punishment has a major effect on offenders (Gendreau, 1995). This applies even more strongly to psychopaths, because they have deficits in avoidance learning and are low in anxiety (Cleckley, 1976; Hare, 1995; Lykken, 1995). Thus, for example, offenders with high scores on the PCL-R are particularly at risk of reoffending after a variety of sentences such as imprisonment, parole, and mandatory supervision (Gendreau, Little, & Goggin, 1995; Hart, Kropp, & Hare, 1988; Harpur, Hare, & Hakstian, 1989; Hemphill et al., 1998; Salekin et al., 1996). In comparison with other serious offenders, they also have a higher rate of prior offending and spend the longest proportion of their lives in prison (Bender &

Lösel, 2000; Hemphill et al., 1998). The predictive validity of the PCL-R holds for various types of offending and particularly for violent recidivism (Harris, Rice, & Quinsey, 1993; Hemphill et al., 1998; Salekin et al., 1996; Serin, 1996). Of course, this predictive validity is particularly due to its second factor that includes items on antisocial life-style. However, it is not only the criminal history but also the interpersonal and affective characteristics represented in the first factor that contribute here (Hemphill et al., 1998).

This body of research suggests that the traditional measures of the penal system or "punishment smarter" strategies are less successful for psychopaths than for other offenders. There may be only one exception: long-term selective incapacitation such as the Californian rule of "Three strikes and you're out." Although such an approach may contribute to the protection of the public, it is confronted with ethical, legal, empirical, and practical problems. For example: (a) According to the principle of just desert punishment, the length of incarceration must be in proportion to the seriousness of the offense (von Hirsch, 1993). (b) Although the PCL-R is a relatively good predictor of violent recidivism or dangerousness, the respective correlations are still too moderate for avoiding high rates of false positives. (c) Because the criminal careers of psychopaths fade out relatively late in life (Hare, McPherson, & Forth, 1988), selective incapacitation would be necessary for very long time periods. (d) Imprisonment is extremely expensive and less cost-effective than other measures of intervention (Greenwood, Model, Rydell, & Chiesa, 1996; Skolnick, 1994). (e) Many psychopaths do not engage in serious criminality although they do a lot of harm to other people. Such arguments do not contradict the use of psychopathy as a marker in decisions on custody and level of security. However, in the long run, expanded imprisonment may not only come into conflict with basic values of humanity but can also reduce investments in education and thus indirectly lead to crime in society.

2.4. Pharmacological treatment

Biological factors and biosocial interactions play an important role in persistent violence and psychopathy (e.g., Hare, 1995; Raine et al., 1997; see, also, Raine, this volume). Thus, pharmacological treatment may be a promising approach. It can be related to Gray's (1982, 1987) concept of brain function. Gray distinguishes (a) the mesolimbic dopamine system, activated by conditioned rewards or withdrawal of negative reinforcement stimuli (behavioral activation system or approach system; BAS); (b) the septo-hippocampal system with serotonin and norepinephrine (noradrenaline) as transmitters, activated by conditioned punishment and new stimuli (behavioral inhibition system; BIS); (c) amygdala, activated by aversive stimuli like extreme noise or unexpected attacks (fight/flight system). Theories of psychopathy suggest a relative dominance of the BAS over the BIS (e.g., Newman & Wallace, 1993b; Quay, 1993). This dominance of BAS results in impulsive and aggressive behavior, low frustration tolerance, reduced capacity for passive avoidance learning, and the like that are features of the psychopathic personality. Because impulsive aggression seems to correlate with a diminished serotonergic and possibly noradrenergic functioning but no increased dopaminergic activity (Markowitz & Coccaro, 1995), the dominance of BAS primarily may result from a weak BIS rather than an overactive BAS (Quay, 1993). Related hypotheses refer to problems in evaluation and the monitoring of responses (Newman, 1998), functional deficits in the medial area of the prefrontal cortex (Damasio, 1994; Jurado & Junque, 1996; Lapierre, Braun, & Hodgins, 1995; Raine, 1997), and a lack of violence inhibition mechanisms (Blair, 1995). Unfortunately, most pharmacological studies on the treatment of antisocial behavior are not based on such concepts. They often address vaguely defined psychopathy and patients who have another diagnosis of personality disorder or psychiatric syndromes (Dolan & Coid, 1993; Tardiff, 1992).

Sedative drugs, for example, are contra-indicated in psychopathic personalities (Dolan & Coid, 1993; Tardiff, 1992). Treatment with benzodiazepines may result in behavioral dyscontrol and aggression (Browne et al., 1993). Lithium, however, can be thought of as operating to increase BIS inhibition of BAS. This has been supported partly in the treatment of patients with impulsive and aggressive outbursts or with borderline personality disorders (e.g., Dolan & Coid, 1993; Goldberg, 1989). Less is known about its use in treating antisocial personalities (Wistedt, Helldin, Omerov, & Palmstierna, 1994). Because lithium bears a risk of intoxication and other negative side effects, it is not particularly appropriate (Hollweg & Nedopil, 1997; Markovitz, 1995).

As dopamine receptor blockers, *neuroleptics* can be expected to dampen BAS activity. There seems to be some indication in favor of low-dose neuroleptic therapy in agitated antisocial persons who also show schizotypal features (Soloff et al., 1986; Wistedt et al., 1994).

A more promising approach is suggested by treatment with *serotonin reuptake inhibitors* (SRIs; e.g., fluoxetine, sertraline). For example, in a prospective study with sertraline, Kavoussi, Liu, and Coccaro (1994) found relatively positive effects on the impulsive-aggressive behavior of personality disordered patients. Markovitz, Calabrese, Schulz, and Meltzer (1991) noted positive outcomes in a study of fluoxetine. However, more controlled studies are necessary, in particular, with respect to precisely defined psychopathy.

In the field of sexual offending, *testosterone antagonists* like cyproterone acetate and medroxyprogesterone acetate are applied with some success (Gottesman & Schubert, 1993; Hall, 1995). Because testosterone is related not only to sexuality in the narrow sense but also to dominant, aggressive, and impulsive behavior, antiandrogens would fit the versatile antisociality of many sex offenders and also the psychopaths among them. However, it is not clear whether a high testosterone level is a cause or consequence of aggressive dominance (Archer, 1991). In addition, the testosterone levels of most sex offenders are in the normal range (Barbaree, 1990; Hucker & Bain, 1990). Hormones influence the monoamine receptors. Thus, decreased serotonin (5-HT) may disinhibit or promote sexual behavior, whereas decreased central dopaminergic functioning reduces motivation, including male sexual behavior (Kafka, 1995). Hormones and monoamine neurotransmitters interact in a dynamic fashion that determines the form and intensity of drive (Everitt, 1983). Thus, the use of selective SRIs can be a promising addition to the pharmacotherapy of sexual offenders with antiandrogens (Kafka & Prentky, 1992).

These and other results show that there is not yet one specific drug for the treatment of aggression, impulsivity, and related disorders (Browne et al., 1993; Markovitz, 1995; Wistedt et al., 1994). Furthermore, we do not know whether pharmacotherapy is specifically adequate for psychopaths. However, if potential comorbidities are addressed carefully, pharmacotherapy shows some promise for the future (Dolan & Coid, 1993). For legal and medical reasons, pharmacological treatment will rarely be the first and only choice. However, the successful combination of cognitive-behavioral therapy and pharmacotherapy in the treatment of depression can function as a model. Perhaps, brain imaging research on psychopathy may contribute to further modes of biological intervention (see Raine & Liu, 1998; Raine, this volume).

3. CONCLUSIONS AND PRACTICAL PERSPECTIVES

This brief review discloses strong reasons for striving toward effective management and treatment of psychopathy. It also underlines the clear lack of controlled research on this topic. According to our present knowledge, *psychotherapeutic, educational, and similar psychosocial programs* seem to be partly adequate and partly inadequate. Most promising are intensive, structured, cognitive-behavioral, and multimodal programs that fit the individual criminogenic needs and learning styles of the offenders. Relatively low structured, nondirective, psychotherapeutic, and psychodynamic programs seem to have no effects or sometimes negative outcomes in comparison with untreated control groups. *Therapeutic communities, milieu therapy, and social therapy* must also be evaluated in a differentiated way. Relatively permissive, low-structured milieu therapy and classical therapeutic communities that rely mainly on social group processes and self-direction of the inmates show no or even negative effects. In contrast, well-structured, hierarchical therapeutic communities and social-therapeutic prisons seem to be more adequate. This includes, for example, strictly regimented activities, clearly ordered social roles and responsibilities, consistent reward or punishment of good or bad conduct, and a stepwise contact with the world outside depending on behavioral progress and risk-assessment. *Pure punishment, deterrence, and formal justice reactions* may protect society as long as offenders are incarcerated. However, basic research on the psychopathic personality as well as program evaluation studies show that this group is least influenced by measures of punishment and deterrence. Formal variations in the penal justice system, modern alternative sanctions, and "punishment smarter" strategies also do not seem to be promising in these cases. *Pharmacological treatment* can address deficits in the behavior inhibition system. Depending on respective comorbidities, various modes of such treatment may be indicated for some subgroups. Although more controlled studies are needed, treatment with serotonin re-uptake inhibitors and (in some subgroups of sex offenders) testosterone antagonists seems to be most promising.

In conclusion, evaluation research as well as practical experience do not yet reveal a "royal path" leading to an effective treatment and management of psychopaths. However, there arc empirically based signposts for adequate programs that should be implemented and evaluated carefully at various sites. From a realistic perspective, programs should not attempt to change the core personality of psychopaths. However, interventions should lead to experiences, learning processes, and skills that enable these individuals to express and control their basic personality dispositions in a noncriminal way (Hare, 1995; 1999). According to Lösel (1998), relatively promising programs for psychopaths may contain the following principles:

3.1. Theoretically sound conceptualization

Interventions should not be based on specific schools of psychotherapy but on what is empirically known about psychopathy and criminal behavior. A majority of programs that have proven to be most appropriate for various groups of offenders are based on cognitive social learning theory (Andrews & Bonta, 1994). These approaches seem to be transferable to the psychopathic clientele. However, such concepts must be supplemented by neurophysiological findings on psychopathy. A sound theoretical approach also needs to consider comorbidities (e.g., alcohol dependence), individual kinds of offense (e.g., violence, sexual), and eventual personality subtypes (e.g., in secondary psychopaths). Within a broader evaluation theory (Chen, 1989), an adequate treatment concept must include indicators of goal attainment. For example, working on specific psychopathic thinking patterns, teaching skills for self-control and noncriminal behavior, or reducing alcohol abuse are more adequate than unrealistic aims of changing the core personality. Last but not least, such a theoretical concept should address the risks of abusing program elements.

3.2. Thorough dynamic assessment of the offender

Any intervention must be based on and continuously evaluated through accurate and detailed assessments of the respective case. This includes data on the personality disorder, clinical syndromes, and specific behavioral problems (Dolan & Coid, 1993). Standardized measures of psychopathy like the PCL-R should be used as a central marker. Other instruments such as the SHAPS (Blackburn, 1987), LSI-R (Andrews & Bonta, 1994), VRAG (Quinsey, Harris, Rice, & Cormier, 1998) or more specific scales like the SONAR (Hanson & Harris, 2000) or SV-20 (Boer, Hart, Kropp, & Webster, 1997) are further indicated. Detailed assessments of their more or less superficial treatment motivation and specific kinds of offense are also of interest. Such offense-specific information may provide insight into the links between the psychopathic core personality and specific risks of reoffending. As far as possible, dynamic assessment must rely on multiple sources, objective behavioral indicators, and never the psychopath's verbalization alone.

3.3. Intensive level of service and dosage

Psychopaths have a regular need for an intensive level of service and not short-term programs. Because they are frequently persistent offenders, most interventions will take place in prisons, forensic hospitals, or other institutional settings with a high level of security (Hemphill et al., 1998). Developing at least some motivation for change and testing objective progress in behavior takes a rather long time. Collaboration should be forced by a very cautious delivering of gratifications. Thus, a successful program will need more time than the treatment of most other offenders. High program dosage and a longer duration of treatment have been repeatedly associated with less failures in serious offenders (Cullen, 1997; Dolan, 1997; Lipsey & Wilson, 1998). Early termination due to superficial adaptation of psychopaths must be avoided. As psychopaths often drop out of programs due to their misbehavior or motivational problems (Jones, 1997; Rice et al., 1992), irregular termination should be avoided as far as possible and contain no positive rewards.

3.4. Clearly structured and controlled setting

The institutional context must avoid reinforcing the typical manipulations, blamings, negotiations, and so forth of psychopaths. Thus, a well-structured and supervised setting is indicated. If possible, the therapeutic institution or department should be separate (Hare, 1999; Lösel & Egg, 1997). However, it should not concentrate only on psychopaths or otherwise worst cases. Strict and clear rules, regulations, rights, duties, and responsibilities must be implemented and controlled consistently. These include, for example, differentiated gratifications and their withdrawal in the case of transgression (specific leisure programs, visits, work outside, day pass, or holidays). Regulations should be fixed in advance to avoid the traps in the interpersonal style of psychopaths. Such structures may reduce the opportunities for manipulative tendencies. They can help also psychopaths to monitor and evaluate their responses (Newman, 1998). Last but not least, the staff and other inmates are better protected against attempts to obtain environmental control.

3.5. Positive institutional climate and regime

Although a firm and consistent staff behavior is particularly necessary for the treatment of psychopathy, the institutional regime must be basically sensitive, constructive, and supportive (Porporino & Baylis, 1993; Woodward, 1997). Organizational climate can have rather different influences in otherwise comparable prisons or hospitals (e.g., Andrews & Dowden, 1999; Moos, 1975; Wing, 1993). Because the behavior of psychopaths easily leads to conflicts and interpersonal problems, the positive aspects of a clearly structured regime are at risk of becoming cold and hostile. Thus, the psychopaths' interpersonal style will gain indirect reinforcement. To counteract such tendencies, the institutional climate must be a continuous focus of attention and self-regulation.

3.6. Addressing specific criminogenic needs

Appropriate targeting of criminogenic needs is particularly important (Gendreau, 1995). The individual needs and intermediate targets have to be derived from the dynamic assessment. A central issue in psychopaths is to convince them that their current attitudes and behavior are not in their self-interest (Hare, 1993). Due to their core personality, promoting conscience and empathy are less realistic targets than in other offenders. However, to some degree, it may be possible to shift rewards and costs for activities toward the noncriminal spectrum; to improve delay of gratification; to reduce criminogenic attributions and neutralizations; to train better impulse control and noncriminal problem solving; to reduce alcohol and other dependencies; to learn from attractive, noncriminal role models; or to strengthen monitoring and supervision in the psychopaths' family and everyday environment. As psychopaths are preoccupied with immediate goals and have difficulties in understanding complex and subtle issues (Hare 1995; Kosson, 1996), changes in information processing are very important (Serin & Brown, 1996). Although we should not expect too much in this regard, need-oriented programs have the advantage of concentrating on a limited number of specific objectives. Probably, the recent three-factor model of psychopathy (Cooke & Michie, 1998) may also be useful for a differentiation of needs in specific cases.

3.7. Measures based on the responsivity principle

As in the treatment of nonpsychopathic serious and violent offenders, it is necessary to implement multimodal and cognitive-behavioral programs. They seem to be most appropriate to change the cognitive distortions, denials, minimizations, and so forth (Serin & Kuriychuk, 1994). As the responsivity principle includes matching treatment mode x offender type x staff style, no general package is suggested. However, existing programs or concepts (e.g., Beck & Freeman, 1990; Hare, 1992; Ross & Ross, 1995) are applicable and can be supplemented or accentuated for specific problems (like sexual offending or alcohol problems). As mentioned above, each element of intervention has to be checked to see whether it is susceptible to misuse. Although it is questionable whether psychopaths are able to form at least a rudimentary therapeutic bond, this cannot be denied in principle (Vaillant, 1975). Therefore, matching with an accepting but firm and consistent staff member is also recommended.

3.8. Realizing high program integrity

Lack of integrity is an important cause of reduced effects in potentially successful programs (Andrews & Dowden, 1995; Hollin, 1995; Lösel & Wittmann, 1989). Low integrity may result from having no well-developed treatment concept as well as from deficits in skills, attitudes, and motivation among staff members. Not least, the behavior of psychopaths may weaken program implementation. Thus, monitoring the quality and quantity of the program is necessary. Regular assessments of integrity cannot be used just for improving the general quality of treatment but also for case conferences. On the one hand, they make manipulative actions of psychopaths more transparent. On the other hand, monitoring can help to detect negative attitudes and counter-transferences in specific staff-client relations.

3.9. Thorough selection, training, and supervision of staff

All principles discussed so far require well selected, sensitive, competent, and multidisciplinary staff members. Selection should not just be oriented toward professional qualifications but personality characteristics as well. For example, relatively anxious, apprehensive, verbal-nonpragmatic, or inexperienced young officers could be misplaced in work with psychopaths. Intensive training must contain detailed knowledge on psychopathy and its management. Continous supervision is relevant for improving professional skills and attitudes on the job (Woodward, 1997). It is also necessary to avoid typical inconsistencies or destructive interpersonal processes in work with psychopaths, for example: (a) battling to win, (b) becoming the advocate, (c) believing what you hear, (d) fearing manipulations, and (e) becoming fascinated (Doren, 1987). Finding the right path between naive trust and disappointed cynicism is very important. This must be encouraged by social support from the agency and community (Andrews, 1995; Roberts, 1995).

3.10. Neutralization of unfavorable social networks and group processes

Deviant peers are modeling and reinforcing influences for antisocial behavior (e.g., Elliott, Huizinga, & Menard, 1989; Thornberry, 1998). Therefore, appropriate programs should try to neutralize these networks. Unfortunately, correctional institutions and forensic hospitals promote unfavorable peer influences through the concentration of individuals with similar problems. Although psychopaths are not closely related to the group, they are influential because of their glibness, manipulation, institutional experience, and so forth. Frequently, they may take over central roles in housekeeping, merchandising, smuggling, or gambling (Hürlimann, 1993). Staff must be aware of such social processes and counteract exploitative relationships through an adequate allocation of inmates. Groups should also develop explicit behavior norms. Here, principles from structured therapeutic communities can be relevant (Wexler, 1997). Relatively firm and cooperative inmates can also adopt an important role in confronting the psychopath with reality. Sometimes, they may function as a kind of co-trainer.

3.11. Strengthening natural protective factors

Most research and practice on the treatment of antisociality is oriented primarily toward risks. However, studies on the natural history of antisocial behavior reveal processes of resilience and desistance that are linked to the protective functions of individual or social resources (e.g., Lösel & Bender, in press). Such protective processes are often similar to those in successful treatment. Like professional interventions, they can help to create turning points in a criminal career. As psychopaths are unsteady, there often will be a lack of protective resources in everyday life. A firm and consistent partner, an "authoritative" climate at work, or specific competencies and talents may have such a function (e.g., Lösel & Bliesener, 1994; Rutter, 1990; Werner &

Smith, 1992). Program staff should try to figure out and strengthen potential protective resources that counteract manipulation and criminogenic social relations after release (e.g., Ditchfield, 1994; Motiuk, 1995).

3.12. Controlled aftercare and relapse prevention

Treatment of antisocial behavior often has only surface or short-term effects. This is particularly likely for personality-disordered offenders (Cullen, 1997). As research on sex offenders and substance abusers has shown, relapse prevention and aftercare are essential for more long-term outcomes (Annis, 1986; Laws, 1999). Released psychopaths should be controlled and supervised regularly to ensure that positive changes are maintained (Serin, 1995). This also includes a thorough assessment of potential abuse of skills acquired during the treatment program. Again, assessment should not rely on information from the subject, but include objective data, work records, and information from others. In some cases, electronic monitoring may be included. The diagnostic component should be combined with additional interventions. Probation officers, social workers, or other staff must be familiar with the facts about psychopathy. Networking between services should be coordinated closely to reduce manipulation. Naturally, all this must be enforced legally.

3.13. Systematic program evaluation

The increased theoretical and practical knowledge on the management and treatment of psychopaths must be tested continuously in methodologically sound program evaluations. Respective studies should not just address whole institutions such as therapeutic communities or social-therapeutic prisons. In these cases, we often do not know enough about replicable processes that are essential for success. On the other hand, it remains unclear why a program fails (Lösel, 1995). Therefore, comprehensive evaluations should include studies of specific program elements and modules. At this level, it is also easier to realize equivalent untreated or waiting control groups. However, evaluation should also address the more complex, multimodal, climatic, and institutional issues of intervention. Here, systematic assessment of process data may give us some information on correlates of success or failure (e.g., Ortmann, 2000).

3.14. Early prevention and intervention

Although the diagnosis of psychopathy and antisocial personality disorder is restricted to adulthood,. there is growing evidence of precursors in childhood and adolescence (Frick, 1998; Forth & Burke, 1998; Lyman, 1996; Moffitt, 1993). For example, Frick (1998) assessed a callous-unemotional subgroup of children with conduct disorders who even misbehaved under conditions of good parenting. Studies on early starting, persistent antisociality reveal a cumulative risk or snowball effect of various bio-psycho-social factors (Lösel & Bender, in press; Yoshikawa, 1994). Against this background, it seems most promising to intervene in fledgling psychopathy before too many risks have cumulated. Reviews suggest that early prevention can be successful (Farrington & Welsh, 1999; Tremblay & Craig, 1995). Successful measures for children at-risk must include elements for improving cognitive and social competencies and reducing impulsivity and attention deficits. However, child programs often do not have a long-term impact (e.g., Beelmann, Pfingsten, & Lösel, 1994). Therefore, they must be accompanied by measures that improve parenting behavior as well (e.g., Patterson, Reid, & Dishion, 1992). Multimodal, intensive, and early starting programs seem to be particularly promising (Lösel, Beelmann, & Stemmler, 1998; Tremblay & Craig, 1995). However, as in the treatment of adult psychopaths, there is still a lack of well-controlled early prevention studies.

3.15. Reducing societal reinforcement

Cultural factors can serve either to suppress or to reinforce the expression of psychopathic behavior (Cooke, 1997; Hare, 1993). In current business life, for example, traditional rules and relations break down rapidly, controls loosen up, organizations become highly dynamic, and managers must take greater risks (Babiak, 1996). At least temporarily, such transitions provide a platform for manipulation, deception, and other psychopathic behavior. Perhaps, emphasis on shareholder value, globalization, modern mobility, and anonymous electronic communication may have a similar effect by reducing social bonds and responsibilities. In private life, long-term relationships become less frequent. Mass media emphasize sensation seeking, short-term oriented lifestyles, and superficial impression making. In television and movies, nuances of social relationships, emotionality, and language are overwhelmed by pure action, aggression, and role stereotypes. Naturally, such factors are not causes of psychopathy. However, we must also address societal processes that may contribute to its behavioral expression.

As the practice of any intervention is related closely to legal and other local, national, and cultural issues, internationally comparative developments and evaluations of programs for psychopaths would be particularly worthwhile.

REFERENCES

Aichhorn, A. (1957): *Verwahrloste Jugend* (4th ed.), Stuttgart, Huber.

Andrews, D. (1995): "The psychology of criminal conduct and effective treatment", in J. McGuire (Ed.), *What works: Reducing reoffending*,. Chichester, Wiley, pp. 35-62.

Andrews, D. A. & Bonta, J. (1994): *The psychology of criminal conduct*, Cincinatti OH,

Anderson.

Andrews, D. A.; Zinger, I.; Hoge, R. D.; Bonta, J.; Gendreau, P. & Cullen, F. T. (1990): "Does correctional treatment work? A clinically-relevant and psychologically informed meta-analysis", *Criminology*, 28, pp. 369-404.

Annis, H. (1986): "A relapse prevention model for treatment of alcoholics", in W. E. Miller & N. Heather (Eds.), *Treating addictive behaviors*, New York, Plenum, pp. 407-435.

Archer, J. (1991): "The influence of testosterone on human aggression", *British Journal of Psychology*, 82, pp. 1-28.

Babiak, P. (1996): "Psychopathic manipulation in organizations: pawns, patrons, and patsies", *Issues in Criminological and Legal Psychology*, 24, pp. 12-17.

Barbaree, H. E. (1990): "Stimulus control of sexual arousal: Its role in sexual assault", in W. L. Marshall, D. R. Laws & H. E. Barbaree (Eds.), *Handbook of sexual assault: Issues, theories, and treatment of the offender*, New York, Plenum, pp. 115-142.

Beck, A. T. & Freeman, A. (1990): *Cognitive therapy of personality disorders*, New York, Guilford Press.

Beelmann, A.; Pfingsten, U. & Lösel, F. (1994): "Effects of training social competence in children: A meta-analysis of recent evaluation studies", *Journal of Clinical Child Psychology*, 23, pp. 260-271.

Blackburn, R. (1993): "Clinical programs with psychopaths", in K. Howells & C. R. Hollin (Eds.), *Clinical approaches to mentally disordered offenders*, Chichester, Wiley, pp. 179-208.

Boer, D. P.; Hart, S. D.; Kropp, P. R. & Webster, C. (1997): *Manual for the Sexual Violence Risk-20. Professional guidelines for assessing risk of sexual violence*, Burnaby CAN, The Mental Health, Law, and Policy Institute, Simon Fraser University.

Brennan, P. A. & Mednick, S. A. (1994): "Evidence for the adaptation of a learning theory approach to criminal deterrence: A preliminary study", in E. Weitekamp & H.-J. Kerner (Eds.), *Cross-national longitudinal research on human development and criminal behavior*, Dordrecht, Kluwer, pp. 371-379.

Browne, F.; Gudjonsson, G.; Gunn, J.; Rix, G.; Sohn, L. & Taylor, P. J. (1993): "Principles of treatment of the mentally ill offender", in J. Gunn & P. Taylor (Eds.), *Forensic psychiatry: Clinical, legal and ethical issues*, Oxford, Butterworth-Heinemann, pp. 646-690.

Chen, H. T. (1989): *Theory-driven evaluations*, Newbury Park CA, Sage.

Cleckley, H. (1976): *The mask of sanity* (5th ed.), St. Louis MO, Mosby.

Cooke, D. J. (1989): "Containing violent prisoners: An analysis of the Barlinnie Special Unit", *British Journal of Criminology*, 29, pp. 129-143.

Cooke, D. J. (1997a): "Psychopaths: oversexed, overplayed but not over here?", *Criminal Behaviour and Mental Health*, 7, pp. 3-11.

Cooke, D. J. (1997b): "The Barlinnie Special Unit: The rise and fall of a therapeutic experiment", in E. Cullen; L. Jones & R. Woodward (Eds.), *Therapeutic communities for offenders*, Chichester, Wiley, pp. 101-120.

Cooke, D. J. & Michie, C. (1998): "Psychopathy: Exploring the hierarchical structure", Paper presented at the 8th European Conference on Psychology and Law, September 2-5, Krakow, Polonia.

Cullen, E. (1994): "Grendon: the therapeutic prison that works", *Journal of Therapeutic Communities*, 15, 4.

Cullen, E. (1997): "Can a prison be a therapeutic community? The Grendon template", in E. Cullen, L. Jones & R. Woodward (Eds.), *Therapeutic communities for offenders*, Chichester, Wiley, pp. 75-99.

Ditchfield, J. (1994): "Family ties and recidivism: Main findings of the literature", *Research Bulletin of the Home of Office Research and Statistics Department*, 36, pp. 1-9.

Dolan, B. (1997): "A community based TC: The Henderson hospital", in E. Cullen, L. Jones

& R. Woodward (Eds.), *Therapeutic communities for offenders*, Chichester, Wiley, pp. 47-74.

Dolan, B. & Coid, J. (1993): *Psychopathic and antisocial personality disorders*, London, Gaskell.

Dolan, B. M.; Evans, C. D. & Wilson, J. (1992): "Therapeutic community treatment for personality disordered adults: Changes in neurotic symptomatology on follow-up", *International Journal of Social Psychiatry*, 38, pp. 243-250.

Doren, D. M. (1987): *Understanding and treating the psychopath*, Toronto, Wiley.

Eissler, K. R. (1949): "Some problems of delinquency", in K. R. Eissler (Ed.), *Searchlights on delinquency*, New York, International Universities Press, pp. 3-25.

Elliott, D. S.; Huizinga, D. & Menard, S. (1989): *Multiple problem youth*, New York, Springer.

Esteban, C.; Garrido, V. & Molero, C. (1995): *The effectiveness of treatment of psychopathy: A meta-analysis*, Paper presented at the NATO Advanced Study Institute on Psychopathy, November 1996, Alvør, Portugal.

Everitt, B. J. (1983): "Monoamines and the control of sexual behavior", *Psychology and Medicine*, 13, pp. 715-720.

Farrington, D. P. & Welsh, B. (1999): "Delinquency prevention using family-based interventions", *Children and Society*, 13, in press.

Frick, P. J. (1998): "Callous-unemotional traits and conduct problems: Applying the two-factor model of psychopathy to children", in D. J. Cooke, A. E. Forth & R. D. Hare (Eds.), *Psychopathy: Theory, research and implications for society*, Dordrecht, Kluwer, pp. 161-187.

Genders, E. & Player, E. (1995): *Grendon: A study of a therapeutic prison*, Oxford, Clarendon Press.

Gendreau, P. (1995): "The principles of effective intervention with offenders", in A. J. Harland (Ed.), *Choosing correctional options that work: Defining the demand and evaluating the supply*, Thousand Oaks CA, Sage.

Gendreau, P. & Goggin, C. (1996): "Principles of effective programming", *Forum on Corrections Research*, 8(3), pp. 38-41.

Gendreau, P.; Little, T. & Goggin, C. (1995): *A meta-analysis of the predictors of adult offender recidivism: Assessment guidelines for classification and treatment*, Ottawa, Corrections Branch, Ministry Secretariat, Solicitor General of Canada.

Gendreau, P.; Paparozzi, M.; Little, T. & Goddard, M. (1993): "Does 'punishment smarter' work? An assessment of the new generation of alternative sanctions in probation", *Forum on Corrections Research*, 5, pp. 31-34.

Gendreau, P. & Ross, R.R. (1987): "Revivication of rehabilitation: Evidence from the 1980s", *Justice Quarterly*, 4, pp. 349-407.

Goldberg, S. C. (1989): "Lithium in the treatment of borderline personality disorder", *Pharmacological Bulletin*, 25, pp. 550-555.

Gottesman, H. G. & Schubert, D. S. P. (1993): "Low-dose oral medroxyprogesterone acetate in the management of paraphilias", *Journal of Clinical Psychiatry*, 54, pp. 182-187.

Gray, J. A. (1982): *The neuropsychology of anxiety: An enquiry into the function of the septo-hippocampal system*, New York, Oxford University Press.

Gray, J. A. (1987): *The psychology of fear and stress*, New York, Cambridge University Press.

Greenwood, P. W.; Model, K. E.; Rydell, C. P. & Chiesa, J. (1996): *Diverting children from a life to crime: Measuring costs and benefits*, Santa Monica CA, Rand Corporation.

Gunn, J.; Robertson, G. & Dell, S. (1978): *Psychiatric aspects of imprisonment*, London, Academic Press.

Hall, G. C. N. (1995): "Sexual offender recidivism revisited: A meta-analysis of recent treatment studies", *Journal of Consulting and Clinical Psychology*, 63, 5, pp. 802-809.

Hare, R. D. (1991): *The Hare Psychopathy Checklist-Revised*, Toronto, Ontario, Multi-Health Systems.

Hare, F. (1992): *A model program for offenders at high risk for violence*, Ottawa, Correctional Service of Canada.

Hare, R. D. (1993): *Without conscience: The disturbing world of the psychopaths among us*, New York, Simon & Schuster.

Hare, R. D . (1995): "Psychopathy: A clinical construct whose time has come", *Criminal Justice and Behavior*, 23, 25-54.

Hare, R. D.; McPherson, L. E. & Forth, A. E. (1988): "Male psychopaths and their criminal careers", *Journal of Consulting and Clinical Psychology*, 56, pp. 710-714.

Harpur, T. J.; Hare, R. D. & Hakstian, A. R. (1989): "Two-factor conceptualization of psychopathy: Construct validity and assessment implications", *Psychological Assessment: A Journal of Consulting and Clinical Psychology*, 1, 6-17.

Harris, G. T.; Rice, M. E. & Cormier, C.A. (1991): "Psychopathy and violent recidivism", *Law and Human Behavior*, 15, pp. 625-637.

Harris, G. T.; Rice, M. E. & Quinsey, V. L. (1993): "Violent recidivism of mentally disordered offenders: The development of a statistical prediction instrument", *Criminal Justice and Behavior*, 20, pp. 315-335.

Harris, G. T.; Rice, M. E. & Quinsey, V. L. (1994): "Psychopathy as a taxon: Evidence that psychopaths are a discrete class", *Journal of Consulting and Clinical Psychology*, 62, pp. 387-397.

Hart, S. D.; Kropp, P. R. & Hare, R. D. (1988): "Performance of male psychopaths following conditional release from prison", *Journal of Consulting and Clinical Psychology*, 56, pp. 227-232.

Hemphill, J. F. & Hare, R. D. (1996): "Psychopathy Checklist factor scores and recidivism", *Issues in Criminological and Legal Psychology*, 24, pp. 68-73.

Hollin, C. R. (1995): "The meaning and implications of 'programme integrity'", in J. McGuire (Ed.), *What works: Reducing reoffending*, Chichester, Wiley, pp. 195-208.

Hollweg, M. & Nedopil, N. (1997): "Die pharmokologische Behandlung aggressiv-impulsiven Verhaltens", *Psycho*, 23, pp. 308-318.

Hucker, S. J. & Bain, J. (1990): "Androgenic hormones and sexual assault", in W. L. Marshall, D. R. Laws & H. E. Barbaree (Eds.), *Handbook of sexual assault*, New York, Plenum Press, pp. 93-102.

Hürlimann, M. (1993): *Führer und Einflussfaktoren in der Subkultur des Strafvollzugs*, Pfaffenweiler, Centaurus.

Jones, L. (1997): "Developing models for managing treatment integrity and efficacy in a prison-based TC: The Max Glatt Centre", in E. Cullen, L. Jones & R. Woodward (Eds.), *Therapeutic communities for offenders*, Chichester, Wiley, pp. 121-157.

Junger-Tas, J. (1993): "Alternatives to prison: myth and reality", in NISCALE (Ed.), *Report on the workshop on criminality and law enforcement*, Leiden, The Netherlands Institute for the Study of Criminality and Law Enforcement, pp. 104-131.

Kafka, M. P. (1995): "Sexual impulsivity", in E. Hollander & D. J. Stein (Eds.), *Impulsivity and aggression*, Chichester, Wiley, pp. 201-228.

Kafka, M. P. & Prentky, R. (1992): "Fluoxetine treatment of nonparaphilic sexual addictions and paraphilias in men", *Journal of Clinical Psychiatry*, 53, pp. 351-358.

Kavoussi, R. J.; Liu, L. & Coccaro, E. F. (1994): "An open trial of sertraline in personality disordered patients with impulsive aggression", *Journal of Clinical Psychiatry*, 55, pp. 137-141.

Kosson, D. S. (1996): "Psychopathic offenders display performance deficits but not overfocusing under dual-task conditions of unequal priority", *Issues in Criminological and Legal Psychology*, 24, pp. 82-89.

Laws, D. R. (1989): *Relapse prevention with sex offenders*, New York, Guilford Press.

Lapierre, D.; Braun, C. M. & Hodgins, S. (1995): "Ventral frontal deficits in psychopathy: Neuropsychological test findings", *Neuropsychologia*, 33, pp. 139-151.

Lipsey, M. W. (1992a): "Juvenile delinquency treatment: A meta-analytic inquiry into variability of effects", in T. D. Cook, H. Cooper, D. S. Cordray, H. Hartmann, L. V. Hedges, R. L. Light, T. A. Louis & F. Mosteller (Eds.), *Meta-analysis for explanation*, New York, Russell Sage Foundation, pp. 83-127.

Lipsey, M. W. (1992b): "The effect of treatment on juvenile delinquents: Results from meta-analysis", in F. Lösel, D. Bender & T. Bliesener (Eds.), *Psychology and law: International perspectives*, Berlin, De Gruyter, pp. 131-143.

Lipsey, M. W. & Wilson, D. B. (1998): "Effective intervention for serious juvenile offenders", in R. Loeber and D. P. Farrington (Eds.), *Serious and violent juvenile offenders*, Thousand Oaks CA, Sage, pp. 313-345.

Loeber, R.; Farrington, D. P. & Waschbusch, D. A. (1998): "Serious and violent juvenile offenders", in R. Loeber & D.P. Farrington (Eds.), *Serious and violent juvenile offenders*, Thousand Oaks CA, Sage, pp. 13-29.

Logan, C. H.; Gaes, G. G.; Harer, M.; Innes, C. A.; Karacki, L. & Saylor, W. G. (1991): *Can meta-analysis save correctional rehabilitation?* Washington DC, Federal Bureau of Prisons.

Lösel, F. (1995a): "The efficacy of correctional treatment: A review and synthesis of meta-evaluations", in J. McGuire (Ed.), *What works: Reducing reoffending*, Chichester, Wiley, pp. 79-111.

Lösel, F. (1995b): "Increasing consensus in the evaluation of offender rehabilitation? Lessons from research syntheses", *Psychology, Crime and Law*, 2, pp. 19-39.

Lösel, F. (1995c): "Evaluating psychosocial interventions in prison and other penal contexts", in European Committee on Crime Problems (Ed.), *Psychosocial intervention in the criminal justice system*, Strasbourg, Council of Europe, pp. 79-114.

Lösel, F. (1998): "Treatment and management of psychopaths", in D. Cooke, A. Forth & R. D. Hare (Eds.), *Psychopathy: Theory, research, and implications for society*, Dordrecht, Kluwer Academic Publishers, pp. 303-354.

Lösel, F.; Beelmann, A. & Stemmler, M. (1998): *Förderung von Erziehungskompetenzen und sozialen Fertigkeiten in Familien: Eine kombinierte Präventions- und Entwicklungsstudie zu Störungen des Sozialverhaltens*, Projektantrag an das Bundesministerium für Familien, Senioren, Frauen und Jugend. Universität Erlangen-Nürnberg, Institut für Psychologie.

Lösel, F. & Bender, D. (2000): "Protective factors and resilience", in D. P. Farrington & J. Coid (Eds.), *Prevention of adult antisocial behaviour*, Cambridge, Cambridge University Press (in press).

Lösel, F. & Bliesener, T. (1994): "Some high-risk adolescents do not develop conduct problems: A study of protective factors", *International Journal of Behavioral Development*, 4, pp. 753-777.

Lösel, F. & Egg, R. (1997): "Social-therapeutic institutions in Germany: Description and evaluation", in E. Cullen, L. Jones & R. Woodward (Eds.), *Therapeutic communities for offenders*, Chichester: Wiley, pp. 181-203.

Lösel, F. & Wittmann, W. W. (1989): "The relationship of treatment integrity to outcome criteria", in R. F. Conner & M. Hendricks (Eds.), *International innovations in evaluation methodology*, San Francisco, Jossey-Bass, pp. 97-108.

Lykken, D. T. (1995): *The antisocial personalities*, Hillsdale NJ, Lawrence Erlbaum.

Lyman, D. R. (1996): "Early identification of chronic offenders: Who is the fledgling psychopath?", *Psychological Bulletin*, 120, pp. 209-234.

Markovitz, P. (1995): "Pharmacotherapy of impulsivity, aggression, and related disorders", in E. Hollander & D. J. Stein (Eds.), *Impulsivity and aggression*, Chichester, Wiley, pp. 263-287.

Markovitz, P. J.; Calabrese, J. R.; Schulz, S. C. & Meltzer, H. Y. (1991): "Fluoxetine in borderline and schizotypal personality disorder", *American Journal of Psychiatry*, 148, pp. 1064-1067.

Markowitz, P. I. & Coccaro, E. F. (1995): "Biological studies of impulsivity, aggression, and suicidal behavior", in E. Hollander & D. J. Stein (Eds.), *Impulsivity and aggression*, Chichester, Wiley, pp. 71-90.

Marshall, W. L.; Fernandez Y. M.; Hudson, S. M. & Ward, T. (Eds.) (1998): *Sourcebook of treatment programs for sexual offenders*, New York, Plenum Press.

Martinson, R. (1974): "What works? Questions and answers about prison reform", *The Public Interest*, 10, pp. 22-54.

McCord, J. (1978): "A thirty-year follow-up of treatment effects", *American Psychologist*, 33, pp. 284-289.

McCord, W. (1982): *The psychopath and milieu-therapy: A longitudinal study*, New York, Academic Press.

Moffitt, T. E. (1993): "Adolescence-limited and life-course-persistent antisocial behavior: A developmental taxonomy", *Psychological Review*, 4, pp. 674-701.

Moos, R. (1975): *Evaluationg correctional and community settings*, New York, Wiley.

Motiuk, L. L. (1995): "Using familial factors to assess offender risk and need", *Forum on Corrections Research*, 7 (2), pp. 19-22.

Newman, J. P. & Wallace, J. F. (1993b): "Diverse pathways to deficient self-regulation: Implications for disinhibitory psychopathology in children", *Clinical Psychology Review*, 13, pp. 699-720.

Ogloff, J. R. P.; Wong, S. & Greenwood, A. (1990): "Treating criminal psychopaths in a therapeutic community program", *Behavioral Sciences and the Law*, 8, pp. 181-190.

Orlinsky, D. E.; Grawe, K. & Parks, B. K. (1994): "Process and outcome in psychotherapy - noch einmal", in A. E. Bergin & S. L. Garfield (Eds.), *Handbook of psychotherapy and behavior change* (4th ed.), New York, Wiley, pp. 270-376.

Patterson, G. R.; Reid, J. B. & Dishion, T. J. (1992): *Antisocial boys*, Eugene OR, Castalia.

Peat, B. J. & Winfree, L. T. (1992): "Reducing intra-institutional effects of 'prisonization'. A study of a therapeutic community for drug-using inmates", *Criminal Justice and Behavior*, 19, pp. 206-225.

Petersilia, J.; Turner & Dechenes, E. P. (1992): "The costs and effects of intensive supervision for drug offenders", *Federal Probation*, 61, pp. 12-17.

Porporino, F. & Baylis, E. (1993): "Designing a progressive penology: the evolution of Canadian federal correction", *Criminal Behaviour and Mental Health*, 3, pp. 268-289.

Quay, H. C. (1993): "The psychobiology of undersocialized aggressive conduct disorder: A theoretical perspective", *Development and Psychopathology*, 5, pp. 165-180.

Raine, A. (1993): *The psychopathology of crime*, San Diego, Academic Press.

Raine, A. (1997): "Antisocial behavior and psychophysiology: A biosocial perspective and a prefrontal dysfunction hypothesis", in D. M. Stoff, J. Breiling & J. D. Maser (Eds.), *Handbook of antisocial behavior*, New York, Wiley, pp. 289-304.

Raine, A.; Farrington, D. P.; Brennan, P. & Mednick, S. A. (Eds.) (1997): *Biosocial bases of violence*, New York, Plenum Press (in press).

Redondo, S.; Sánchez-Meca, J. & Garrido, V. (1999): "The influence of treatment programmes on the recidivism of juvenile and adult offenders: An European meta-analytic review", *Psychology, Crime and Law*, 5, pp. 251-278.

Redondo, S.; Sánchez-Meca, J. & Garrido, V. (in press): "Crime treatment in Europe: A final view of the century and future perspectives", in J. McGuire (Ed.), *Offender rehabilitation and treatment: Effective programmes and policies to reduce re-offending*, Chichester, Wiley.

Rice, M. E.; Harris, G. T. & Cormier, C.A. (1992): "An evaluation of a maximum security therapeutic community for psychopaths and other mentally disordered offenders", *Law and Human Behavior*, 16, pp. 399-412.

Roberts, C. (1995): "Effective practice and service delivery", in J. McGuire (Ed.), *What works: Reducing reoffending*, Chichester, Wiley, pp. 221-236.

Roberts, J. (1997): "History of the therapeutic community", in E. Cullen, L. Jones & R. Woodward (Eds.), *Therapeutic communities for offenders*, Chichester, Wiley, pp. 3-22.

Robertson, G. & Gunn, J. (1987): "A ten-year follow-up of men discharged from Grendon Prison", *British Journal of Psychiatry*, 151, pp. 674-678.

Ross, R. R. & Ross, B. (Eds.)(1995): *Thinking straight*, Ottawa, Cognitive Centre.

Rowe, D. C. (1994): *The limits of family influence: Genes, experience, and behavior*, New York, Guilford.

Rutter, M. (1990): "Psychosocial resilience and protective mechanisms", in J. Rolf, A. Masten, D. Cicchetti, K. Nuechterlein & S. Weintraub (Eds.), *Risk and protective factors in the development of psychopathology*, Cambridge, Cambridge University Press, pp. 181-214.

Rutter, M.; Giller, H. & Hagell, A. (1998): *Antisocial behavior by young people*, Cambridge UK, Cambridge University Press.

Salekin, R. T.; Rogers, R. & Sewell, K. W. (1996): "A review and meta-analysis of the Psychopathy Checklist and Psychopathy Checklist-Revised: Predictive validity of dangerousness", *Clinical Psychology: Science and Practice*, 3, pp. 203-215.

Serin, R. (1995): "Treatment responsivity in criminal psychopaths", *Forum on Corrections Research*, 7(3), pp. 23-26.

Serin, R. & Brown, S. (1996): "Strategies for enhancing the treatment of violent offenders", *Forum on Corrections Research*, 8(3), pp. 45-48.

Serin, R. C. & Kuriychuk, M. (1994): "Social and cognitive processing deficits in violent offenders: Implications for treatment", *International Journal of Law and Psychiatry*, 17, pp. 431-441.

Skolnick, J. H. (1994): "What not to do about crime", *Criminology*, 33, pp. 1-15.

Soloff, P. H.; George, A.; Nathan, R. S.; Schulz, P. M.; Ulrich, R. F. & Perel, J. M. (1986): "Progress in pharmacotherapy of borderline disorders: A double-blind study of amitriptyline, haloperidol and placebo", *Archives of General Psychiatry*, 43, pp. 691-697.

Tennent, G.; Tennent, D.; Prins, H. & Bedford, A. (1993): "Is psychopathic disorder a treatable condition?", *Medicine, Science, and the Law*, 33, pp. 63-66.

Thornberry, T. P. (1998): "Membership in youth gangs and involvement in serious and violent offending", in R. Loeber & D. P. Farrington (Eds.), *Serious & violent juvenile offenders*, Thousand Oaks CA, Sage, pp. 147-166.

Tremblay, R. E. & Craig, W. M. (1995): "Developmental prevention of crime", in N. Morris & M. Tonry (Eds.), *Building a safer society: Strategic approaches to crime prevention*, Chicago, University of Chicago Press, pp. 151-236.

Vaillant, G. E. (1975): "Sociopathy as a human process. A viewpoint", *Archives of General Psychiatry*, 32, pp. 178-183.

Welsh, B. C. & Farrington, D. P. (1999): "Monetary costs and benefits of crime prevention programs", in M. Tonry (Ed.), *Crime and Justice: A Review of Research*, vol. 25. Chicago IL, University of Chicago Press.

Werner, E. E. & Smith, R. S. (1992): *Overcoming the odds*, Ithaca, Cornell University Press.

Wexler, H. (1997): "Therapeutic communities in American prisons", in E. Cullen, L. Jones & R. Woodward (Eds.), *Therapeutic communities for offenders*, Chichester, Wiley, pp. 161-179.

Wexler, H. K.; Falkin, G. P. & Lipton, D. S. (1990): "Outcome evaluation of a prison therapeutic community for substance abuse treatment", *Criminal Justice and Behavior*, 17, pp. 71-92.

Wing, J. K. (1993): "Institutionalism revisited", *Criminal Behaviour and Mental Health*, 3, pp. 441-451.

Wistedt, B.; Helldin, L.; Omerov, M. & Palmstierna, T. (1994): "Pharmacotherapy for aggressive and violent behaviour: A view of practical management from clinicians", *Criminal Behaviour and Mental Health*, 4, pp. 328-340.

Woodward, R. (1997): "Selection and training of staff for the therapeutic role in the prison setting", in E. Cullen, L. Jones & R. Woodward (Eds.), *Therapeutic communities for offenders*, Chichester, Wiley, pp. 223-252.

Yoshikawa, H. (1994): "Prevention as cumulative protection: Effects of early family support and education on chronic delinquency and its risks", *Psychological Bulletin*, 115, pp. 28-54.

INDEX